MW00992593

ancient way of beauty™

The Art of Japanese Facial Massage

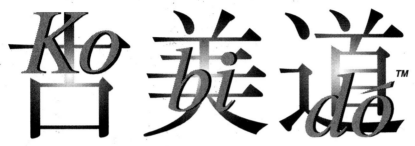

ancient way of beauty™

The Art of Japanese Facial Massage

Popular Edition
taken from: Ko bi do™ - ancient way of beauty™
The Art of Japanese Facial Massage; Professional Edition

Shogo Mochizuki

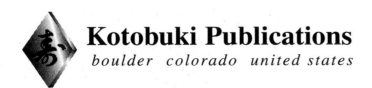

Kotobuki Publications

boulder colorado united states

Ko bi do™: ancient way of beauty™
The Art of Japanese Facial Massage
Popular Edition

Published in the United States by

Kotobuki Publications
P.O. Box 19917
Boulder, CO   80308-2917

ISBN : 1-57615-053-4
Library of Congress Cataloging-in-Publication Data

The author of this book is Shogo Mochizuki.

Copyright © 1999 By Shogo Mochizuki and
James Masamichi Mochizuki-Freeman

NOTE TO THE READER:

> All materials and instructions contained in this book require supervised training by a qualified professional. Authors, publisher, or Japanese Massage and Bodywork Institute are not responsible for the effects of the procedures contained in this book. All matters regarding your health require medical supervision and these materials are not a substitute for qualified care or treatment.

Printed in the United States

First Edition

1   3   5   7   6   4   2

ACKNOWLEDGEMENTS

In the process of creating this book, I have many people to thank. This book would not have been possible without each person's unique contributions. I appreciate their support, and it is my hope that the readers of this book see the value of their contributions of positive energy.

I would like to thank my grandmother for sharing her knowledge and guidance with me and leading me to the study and practice of traditional Japanese medicine and massage. I thank my family members and ancestors who have practiced traditional medicine for over two centuries. I also deeply appreciate my family, particularly my mother and father, who have always provided support.

Thanks to James Yule for his wonderful photographic contributions. Thanks also to Lily Tsong and Megumi Mochizuki for modeling.

Special thanks to Jeffrey Stevens, senior editor of Kotobuki Publications for his valuable contribution.

Also, my deepest appreciation goes out to all of the staff and students of massage schools who have made our workshops possible.

Thanks to many of my friends who have helped in numerous way and the many people who have supported my practice over the years.

Production Staff

Special thanks to the following people and the many others who have been involved with this project over the years.

Inside	*Editor-In-Chief*	• *jeffrey* STEVENS
	Photography	• *james* YULE
	Models	• *lily* TSONG
	Text Editing	• *elizabeth* FLANAGAN
		• *kim* FREEMAN
		• *jeanne* HOENE
		• *kimbo* SNYDER
	Graphics	• *brian* MATHEWS
	Japanese Calligraphy	• *shogo* MOCHIZUKI
Cover	*Design*	• *brian* MATHEWS
	Photography	• *james* YULE
	Models	• *megumi* MOCHIZUKI
		• *lily* TSONG

Special thanks to the following people for the revisions of the 1999 popular edition;

	Text Editing	• *jeffrey* STEVENS
	Text Proofing	• *anne* O'BRIEN
		• *shinji* TSUJI

PREFACE

According to an old Japanese proverb, "A man's face tells everything about him." The face shows the world an individual's physical and psychological state of health as well as featuring glimpses of character and personal history. Being such a unique part of the body, the face one person from another; frequently a person is remembered exclusively by memory of the face alone. The Japanese concept of health defines beauty as an optimal, balanced state of physical, psychological, and spiritual health; the appearance of beauty, often identified solely by the face, is an indicator of this deep state of overall health.

Massage, anma, shiatsu, and other forms of bodywork have become more popular in recent years as ways to help people achieve and enhance the state of healthy beauty and balance. You will find the excellent Japanese facial-massage techniques both easy and beneficial to integrate with other full-body massage methods. For facial practitioners, Japanese facial massage will expand and further your massage repertoire. The Japanese facial-massage concepts come from traditional East Asian medical practices, along with techniques that have been developed and modified from anma (traditional Japanese massage—called anmo in Chinese), the oldest form of massage that originated in ancient China over 5,000 years ago.

Japanese facial massage is one of the best massage techniques I have studied over the years, combining the art and science of massage to enhance health, beauty, and well-being. A good facial massage can always give great relaxation and comfort. I am honored to have the opportunity to share this with you.

Since I completed *Anma: The Art of Japanese Massage*, I decided to compose both a Japanese facial massage and *zoku shin do* textbook to make these practices available to students outside of my classroom.

The early stages for developing this book began in 1992, when I began teaching Japanese facial massage, and I was unable to find any textbooks which provided technical information and practical instructions for the application of those techniques. To teach effectively, I needed to develop a textbook to provide students with the much-needed information. Initially, the professional textbook was thirty pages long, and over time it has grown to include photos and illustrations to become over 420 pages.

In the summer of 1996, I started extracting portions of information from the teaching textbook to create this popular edition, *The Art of Japanese Facial Massage*. I carefully selected techniques that were easy to understand and accessible to anyone who wants to know more about Japanese facial massage, without the technical language and professional emphasis. Over 400 new photographs were used to illustrate the techniques and descriptions in this book. During the summer of 1997, with the contributions of many people, the book was finally completed and is now available to interested persons outside of my classroom. In the Spring of 1999, I revised this textbook to make Japanese facial massage accessible to a wider audience.

My main intention in developing this book has been to explain the techniques of Japanese facial massage as clearly and precisely as possible. In this popular edition, my focus is to reach people who would benefit from learning the techniques of Japanese facial massage. I have selected techniques that are the easiest for a layperson to learn. A few techniques are slightly more advanced but are necessary for a complete facial massage. In addition, most of the technical medical terminology (such as muscle and bone names) are explained in terms easily understood by the layperson. This book provides a better understanding of the foundations of Japanese facial massage and is beneficial for laypeople, as well as offering fresh information for massage therapists, cosmetologists, estheticians, and other beauty and health professionals.

Thanks again to every individual and student who has supported my work over the years. I would also like to thank you, the reader, for your support. I hope you enjoy this volume.

Shogo Mochizuki
Spring 1999

CONTENTS

Chapter 9. Energizing Techniques 115

Chapter 10. Finishing Touch 173

Final Thoughts 185

Index 189

Chapter One

ANCIENT WAY OF BEAUTY™

Long before the times of Jesus and Buddha, rulers in the West valued gold and diamonds and the quest for material wealth. For emperors in the East, it was somewhat different: good health and longevity—even immortality—were the most valuable things to acquire, and the emperors exerted much effort in the quest for them.

Beauty is an important aspect of health and balance: it helps create and maintain optimal health by bringing joy and happiness into an individual's life. Throughout the course of human history, beauty has been a coveted condition, a sign of health and well-being. Recent surveys show that women in the United States spend an average of 360 hours per year in front of the cosmetic mirror—almost one hour per day! It is no surprise that the beauty and cosmetics industry has become a multi-billion dollar enterprise, an empire so rich that the revenues from these industries alone could easily feed the hungry people of the entire world.

In the modern world, especially in the western countries, facial beauty has grown into an obsession. An old Japanese proverb says "one thousand people have one thousand faces." Every face is unique and so characteristically different that people distinguish each other by a quick look to the face. Of course, people desire to improve their most characteristic feature—it is a way of improving self-image.

Japanese facial massage developed to improve one's health and longevity, emphasizing the prevention of problems rather than curing existing ones. When properly administered, it improves one's beauty, removes toxins from the face, and balances *ki*, or life force, to improve overall health.

In Japan, beauty is considered the optimal state of health. Even an attractively-shaped face cannot be beautiful if the person is not well; health and beauty are not separate. Japanese facial massage cannot change the shape of the face, but it certainly can bring about a beautiful, healthy appearance. When a person glows with the radiance of true health, nothing else is necessary for genuine beauty.

Anyone can benefit from Japanese facial massage, from infants and children to men, women, and elders; but perhaps the group that benefits the most is that of women and men over thirty-five. Japanese facial massage is known as one of the best methods of facial care. It does not require any equipment and can be applied anywhere at any time. Unlike facial surgery, Japanese facial massage has no ill side effects.

Japanese facial massage is different from any other system of facial massage. Most methods of facial massage simply work the surface of the face to relax and refresh the tissues. While they do accomplish this to some degree, they are not geared toward more extensive therapy. Japanese facial massage is a profound combination of the traditional Japanese medical concepts and distinct hand-manipulation techniques. It is a branch of Japanese medicine built from the long tradition of diagnostic medicine in the traditions such as anma and acupuncture. From its technical origins in anma, the procedure has reached its present refinement in the last 200 to 300 years within the beauty and cosmetology industry. Today, Japanese facial massage is an independent modality, standing on its own as an area of specialized therapeutic care.

The aim of Japanese facial massage is unique—while Western facial massage addresses the external skin itself, Japanese facial massage is concerned with the condition of skin, subcutaneous musculature, and what is referred to as *ki*, or the life-force energy, often translated as "bioelectricity." Traditionally, the purpose of Japanese facial massage is to work specifically and precisely with the facial meridian and *tsubo* to achieve a balance in the facial skin, the facial muscles, and the related body.

The typical Western massage is a two-stage facial massage of simply cleansing and moisturizing; although this is a relaxing procedure, it is insufficient for actual facial treatment. Japanese facial massage uses three stages: cleansing, moisturizing, and energizing.

The focus of Japanese facial massage is not just to improve facial appearance and to balance *ki* but to also balance psychological conditions. It utilizes traditional Japanese medical concepts such as meridians and *tsubo* to balance and harmonize the condition of internal organs. Important meridians originate and terminate in this region, and there are several points at which *ki* passes from one meridian to another. Massaging the face, very gently stroking the meridians, and applying gentle pressure to certain *tsubo* points can improve *ki* flow. In Japanese facial massage, this stimulation of the meridians and *tsubo* is called the energizing stage. This occurs after the cleansing and moisturizing stages.

In modern times, it is becoming more common to use acupuncture to stimulate the *tsubo* of the face. This activates facial nerves and thus increases the *ki* flow to the face which brings about a natural face-lift effect. However, using the fingertips to activate the *tsubo* for a slightly milder stimulation (in the energizing stage), in combination with the Japanese facial-massage techniques, accomplishes the same effect. Light finger pressure is generally preferable to inserting a needle into the face as with acupuncture, and the results with Japanese facial massage and finger pressure will be similar, if not better, than the natural face-lift response done with acupuncture.

Stimulating *tsubo* by finger pressure is much more effective when the tissue is activated and warmed and the muscles relaxed; the pressure can then be received by the client without muscle resistance. If pressure is applied against a tight or over-contracted facial muscle, the muscle will react against the pressure and frustrate any attempt at therapy. Once the facial tissues are warmed and relaxed, the client will receive pressure with less discomfort, and the overall effect will be better. For this reason, stimulation of *tsubo* is reserved for the third stage of Japanese facial massage, when the tissues are well-prepared and relaxed.

In traditional Japanese and Chinese medicine, the main focus is the prevention of illness rather than the attempted cure of advanced ailments. The oldest-known medical text in the world, *Hung Ti Ni Ching Su Wen*, was written in China over 2,000 years ago, and became the Bible of traditional medicine in East Asia. The main topic of its primary chapters is the prevention of illness; after these sections there follows discussion of specific cures for illnesses, which is given as supplementary information in the event that preventative measures were not taken. The concept of Japanese facial massage is the same. It is designed to help prevent aging and facial problems. It is best to use Japanese facial massage to prevent wrinkles and age spots rather than trying to remove them once they appear.

In Japan, anma—the traditional Japanese massage—has been part of daily life for centuries. In fact, this sort of touch between family members and friends serves to keep people together—it deepens the sense of community. In Japanese families massage is a traditional part of the education parents pass to their children; the assistance that family members can give one another through massage is invaluable in maintaining health and family affection. In western countries, many people are extremely uncomfortable touching others or being touched, even by family members or friends. This does not develop community, this develops isolation and neurosis! I remember, when I was five or six years old, the only way to get extra small change for candy or toys was to give anma to my parents or grandparents, using simple techniques such as percussion to the shoulders and neck or walking on their backs. This was how most people learned anma in Japan. This sort of touch was common enough to be an expected family contribution.

My family has been practicing many forms of traditional Japanese medicine, as well as traditional forms of bodywork (such as anma), for over two centuries. I studied mainly under my grand-mother, who was a very well-known practitioner in Japan. I began studying when I was three years old, beginning with anma, and continuing on to acupuncture two years later.

I first encountered Japanese facial massage when I was four years old and began to accompany my mother to her regular beauty-salon hair appointment. When you go to a beauty salon or barber in Japan, you often receive a neck and facial massage as part of the routine. As I grew up, I continued watching my mother's facial massages every month at the salon and was always curious about the procedure. Later, when I was a teenager, I began studying judo, and massage techniques were included as part of the training. I continued on as an adult and studied a few different styles of facial massage, but nothing was particularly insightful or exceptional about the methods I learned in massage schools.

One day a schoolmate told me about an exceptionally talented facial-massage instructor who was teaching in a beauty school in uptown Tokyo. By that time, facial massage was just facial massage to me, but I changed my viewpoint completely when I studied with her. Her technique was much more precise than the ordinary massage techniques I had learned, and they were designed to fit the particular parts of the face and were based on very rich theory and clinical application. The concepts were far more complex than those used by ordinary massage therapists, and it was obvious how important facial massage of this caliber could be to excellent health. I was completely impressed by her method of Japanese facial massage and I began integrating many of her techniques into my work. But theory and technique were not easy—I actually repeated my lessons two more times to feel that I truly and confidently understood the concepts.

For over 240 years, my family practiced traditional medicine in unswerving adherence to its traditional methods of diagnosis and procedure, and my training was rooted entirely in this tradition until I was a teenager. My family specialized in acupuncture and moxibustion (thermal therapy in which a herb called *moxa* is placed upon the surface of the skin and then ignited), and though I learned and appreciated these traditions, my interest was always in physical manipulation and massage. My family directed me to study with specialists in areas distinct from my family's medical tradition, and I am excited to bring all of these traditional forms of Japanese bodywork to the United States.

Chapter Two

JAPANESE CONCEPT OF HEALTH AND BEAUTY

J apanese facial massage is significantly different from other facial-massage methods. Before I can explain what Japanese facial massage is, I must explain how the Japanese concept of health and beauty differs from the Western concept. The very foundation of Japanese thought on health and beauty is unlike anything in the West. It is important to understand this difference before attempting to practice Japanese methods for attaining or maintaining health and beauty.

The Eastern concept of health and beauty originated in ancient China and has been continually refined up until the present day. Health and longevity have been the most coveted of all things in Asia; beauty has always been attributed to optimal health. In fact, beauty has long been considered the overall reflection of an optimal balance of physical, psychological, and spiritual health. According to the Japanese tradition, beauty arises naturally if a person can bring these three factors into harmony.

Traditional Japanese medicine has developed to prolong natural health and prevent disease. In traditional medical theory, there are four categories of health: death, illness, healthiness, and beauty. Beauty is at the top because it is the radiant condition of robust health. In Japan, beautiful health is the ultimate wealth, and it can be cultivated within each human being, rich or poor.

In the West, since the time of ancient Egypt, tremendous energy has been expended searching for objects of material wealth: gold, precious stones, palaces—anything that itself was beautiful or could be used to acquire beautiful things. But the West has emphasized beauty at the expense of physical, psychological, and spiritual health. As a result,

Western medicine has been developed to repair the body once it has fallen ill. In the West, the concepts of health and beauty are entirely unrelated.

These distinctions largely remain today. After World War II, there was an exchange of culture between the western countries and the eastern countries, and now countries such as Japan are becoming westernized and countries like the United States are absorbing the traditions of the East. The Western view of health and beauty is beginning to accept the rich knowledge of much older traditions; the fact that you are reading a book on Japanese massage proves it!

Perhaps the most important medical discovery from ancient China, and the most profound difference that still exists between Eastern and Western medicine, is the concept and manipulation of *ki* (called "*qi*" or "*chi*" in China). *Ki* is the core of Chinese and Japanese medicine and is an enormous factor in Asian philosophy, poetry, calligraphy, martial arts, religion, and nutrition—virtually all of the traditional arts and sciences. In fact, *ki* is not merely considered the basis of medicine, it is considered the basis of life itself. Yet the West has no similar concept.

For some reason, the West has overlooked its development in the understanding of some of the most essential and natural facets of human health. This is a shame, because bioelectricity itself is not an Asian invention; although *ki* is a Japanese word, it is a universal force, existing at the root of every human being.

A similar thing has happened with meditation. Meditation is a natural human activity that has been an integral part of human life in India, Tibet, China, and Japan for thousands of years, but until this century, it was unknown to the West. Even today, the meditation of the ancients is viewed with suspicion, as something exotic or distinctly Eastern. Western cultures have not cultivated an understanding of meditation any more than *ki*. This is the difficulty Western students must face when they begin to investigate Eastern modalities such as anma and Japanese facial massage.

Traditionally, in Japan, the face is one of the primary parts of the body used for diagnosing the condition of *ki*. Facial problems reveal the particular imbalances of *ki*: an extremely pale facial complexion, for example, often indicates irregular functioning of the stomach. Facial beauty is only possible when the *ki* is balanced, and this is why the Japanese concept equates beauty and health.

Unlike the Western approach to treating facial problems, the Japanese often combine their facial-massage treatments with shiatsu, anma, or acupuncture to treat the entire body. The face receives specialized care, and the techniques of Japanese facial massage ensure that the tissues and muscular systems are carefully worked. The meridians running through the face reveal the condition of the entire body, and a good therapist learns a great deal about the client's health as they give a facial massage; therefore, a Japanese facial treatment is commonly combined with more extensive treatment to the rest of the body.

In the East, treatment takes place much earlier in the health-care process; physicians and allied health professionals use prevention and early diagnosis as the key to robust health. The Japanese tradition holds the view that once symptoms appear, the disease has already reached an advanced stage; the objective of Asian medicine is to discover slight imbalances and treat them well before they develop into diseases and before they begin to spread. In this way, treatment is easier and recovery is much quicker. This is the same procedure used in Japanese facial massage, which aims to prevent the facial problems unnecessarily attributed to age.

In Japan, the majority of people trust the ancient ways of medicine because of the rich historical and cultural tradition behind it. The West has only a few traditional methods of healing based on time-tested remedies; folk medicine is treated with suspicion, as if nothing that happened before the twentieth century has medical value. In Japan, there is a great deal of trust in folk medicine. The centuries-old Japanese facial massage is known to be the best facial care. If there were something better, traditional physicians would have discovered or created it a long time ago, and traditional Japanese facial massage as we know it today would be different.

Westerners tend to believe that good health means the absence of visible symptoms. The appearance of symptoms suddenly reverses a person to the thought that they have suddenly fallen into poor health. There is a myth in the West right now that one can achieve perfect health and fitness. Many westerners obsessively count every gram of fat, record every calorie, and monitor their blood pressure in conjunction with an elaborate exercise routine all in search of this condition of "perfect health."

In Japan, there is no such concept as perfect health. It is accepted that people have inherent irregularities or genetic weaknesses that need to be worked with and supported through preventative care throughout their lives. This is not considered a problem, as it does not prevent radiant, optimal (not "perfect") health. Remember, true health to the Japanese physician is the balance of all twelve internal organs, which brings about a balance of physical, psychological, and spiritual health. The objective of Japanese treatment is to achieve and maintain a balanced state of *ki*, which in turn brings the psychological and spiritual conditions into overall harmony. The West seems to have embraced the idea of instant cures for advanced stages of disease, preferring this to the preventive procedures which monitor the body closely to help it steer away from serious disease and which gradually deepens one's physical, psychological, and spiritual health over an entire lifetime.

Causes of Facial Problems

The Japanese tradition speaks of three factors to consider when dealing with facial problems.

The first one is *so in*, which means "genetic factors." Genetic factors influence the facial skin, and you must consider this when you are treating facial problems. For example, genetic factors cause Asians to have significantly less incidence of freckles than Westerners, and they also cause the darker skin of Equatorial people to better tolerate direct sunshine without burning, whereas many Caucasians burn quickly in direct sunshine. Some people have genetically oily or very dry skin, and some people have heavy facial hair. Genetic factors determine many things.

The next factor is *gai in*, which means "outside factors." Traditionally there are many outside factors which can impact the facial skin—such as extremes of heat, cold, dampness, and dryness. Overexposure to these factors damage the balance of the internal organs, which then impact the condition of the facial skin. Of course, a very dry or humid climate impacts the skin directly, as does prolonged exposure to direct sunshine. But certain facial skin conditions may reflect imbalance in the organs from outside factors. *Gai in* also includes your habitual routines: the quality of diet, occupational stress, lack of exercise; all of these are considered outside factors which impact the health of skin and body.

The third factor is *nai in*, which means "internal factors"—imbalance caused by psychological factors. Emotional balance is directly related to the condition of facial health. In Japanese medical tradition, there are five (some texts describe seven) emotions: sadness, fear, anger, happiness, and worry. Experiencing these states of mind excessively can harm the internal organs, and conversely, excessive emotion can be caused by internal organ imbalances. For example, anger corresponds to the liver. Excessive amounts of anger can damage the liver, which is expressed in the face by an excessively oily complexion and an enlarged end of the nose.

Japanese View of Facial Problems

The two most common facial problems are wrinkles and age spots.

Wrinkles

Wrinkles are divided into three main categories. The first category is that of very fine wrinkles that usually develop around the upper and lower eyelids and mouth and lips. The second category includes the somewhat larger, deeper wrinkles around the outside of the eyes, between the eyebrows, and around the nasolabial crease. The third category comprises very deep wrinkles, often developed along the lower cheek, along the side of the jaw, and around the neck region. Often the first category of wrinkles develops into the second category and then into the third category. It is best to start early in this process to arrest development.

In traditional medical theory, wrinkles are said to be caused by severe imbalances between the internal organs, which brings about water or blood deficiency. Wrinkles are considered *kyo* symptoms and are generally caused by *jitsu* symptoms. It is important to begin treatment when the first category of wrinkles appears. When wrinkles have deepened into the second and third category, the condition becomes very difficult to treat.

Age Spots

Traditionally, Japanese therapists diagnose age spots as an excessive internal dampness that causes the skin to "rust," just as metal rusts when exposed to excessive humidity. Age spots are said to be the result of stagnating bodily fluids—when there is poor blood circulation and poor circulation of bodily fluids, toxins are not adequately flushed from the body. As stagnant liquids pool beneath the skin surface, toxins seep into the skin, causing it to "rust."

Five Common Health Conditions

Japanese medicine and Western medicine differ in their approaches to diagnosis and treatment. Western medicine does not tend to look closely at individual conditions in the manner that Asian medicine does. If three people walk into a Western clinic with mild fevers, stuffed or runny noses, and headaches, they are probably diagnosed as having a cold, are given the same medication, and are told to follow similar procedures for recuperation. The concept here is that three people have the same illness, and that the illness can be treated using a standard procedure. If the procedure works, the symptoms vanish. That is the goal.

Japanese medicine is a highly personalized medicine. If three people arrive at a clinic with similar symptoms, they are diagnosed carefully according to *ki* flow and lifestyle and are given very different treatment. Although the symptoms are the same, it is unlikely that they have the same condition, and therefore it is not possible to prescribe a fixed medication for all three patients on the basis of the symptoms alone. The Japanese system treats the patient, not the illness, and the condition, not the symptoms. Facial massage follows this tradition. For example, dry skin may be caused by lung conditions in one patient and kidney conditions in another patient. The causes for wrinkles and age spots also differ from individual to individual.

The terminology of Western diagnosis is very broad; for example, the term "acne" is typically used to describe an abundance of pimples. Someone is told that they have acne, and they are given medication to treat acne. They take the medication, and when the pimples clear, the acne is said to have been treated.

In Japan, acne is not a condition, it is a symptom, as are wrinkles, age spots, and dry skin. Japanese practitioners are interested in treating the condition that causes pimples, not the pimples themselves. Acne can arise out of a number of conditions (liver conditions, excessive heat in the blood, stomach conditions, etc.). The treatment proceeds according to what particular condition has given rise to the symptom of acne in an individual patient. It is considered useless to treat the acne itself.

With professional Japanese therapists, every patient is treated according to their particular diagnosis. For the beginner, it is good to begin by looking at the five most common conditions of irregularity in health.

1. Blood Deficiency Condition

Japanese traditional medical theory considers blood deficiency to be a situation when there is not enough blood in the body. People with this condition are generally thin and weak, with a pale blue or yellow complexion. This is often accompanied by low blood pressure and bad posture, and the person has little energy. The skin itself seems to lack the firmness of healthy skin. The lips appear whitish or light gray. The fingernails also appear white. When this condition has established itself, it is very easy to develop wrinkles and grey hair. If this condition arises, it can be helpful to avoid consumption of milk and dairy products, raw onions, raw vegetables, and raw fish. Avoid also strong spices, coffee, sugar, alcohol, tobacco, soda, green tea, and barley tea.

2. Poor Circulation of Blood

This is a similar condition to the previous condition. A person with this condition has enough blood, but it is not properly circulating. Often the facial tone appears darkened (blue-black or brownish) and has a doughy, lusterless appearance. The lips and nails also appear to be darkened to a purplish red. The person may often feel chilled in the limbs. This condition is prone to wrinkles and age spots. If this condition arises, avoid consumption of brown rice, soy products (such as tofu and soy milk), milk and dairy products, raw vegetables, and raw fish. Also avoid coffee, sugar, tobacco, and soda.

3. Excessive Heat of Blood

In this condition, there is plenty of well-circulated blood, but there is an excessive amount of heat in the blood. This is generally caused by overconsumption of meat, dairy products, oil, and saturated fats. People with this condition often have high energy, sweat easily, have a red, shiny (oily) complexion, easily become overweight, and anger quickly. They often have high blood pressure. This condition is often accompanied by pimples, loss of hair, and a reddish color to the lips and nails. If this condition arises, avoid consumption of pork and beef, raw garlic, onion, and hot spices. Avoid coffee, sugar, tobacco, and alcohol.

4. Excessive Dampness of Body

This is similar to the condition of poor blood circulation, except that although blood is circulating well, other bodily fluids are not circulating properly. In this condition, the body is often bloated and white. The body gains weight easily, and is prone to fungal infections, such as athlete's foot and yeast infections. Lips are generally white and puffy, and facial tone is white and lusterless. If this condition arises, avoid consumption of all dairy products, brown rice, oily or greasy foods, excessively spicy foods, nuts, soda, and alcohol.

5. Kidney Deficiency

The kidney, a very important organ in traditional Japanese medicine, produces life essence (*sei*), which is the source of will-power. If the kidneys become deficient, symptoms commonly include a dark, pale-bluish face; dark blue-black "bags" beneath the eyes, graying of the hair or premature hair loss, low energy, low sex drive, impotence, and menstrual irregularities. If this condition arises, avoid overconsumption of alcohol. Also, make certain that sleep patterns are regular and sufficient. Finally, avoid consumption of stimulants (such as caffeine, sugar, and salt), and reduce consumption of liquids four hours prior to bedtime.

Chapter Three

WHAT IS JAPANESE FACIAL MASSAGE?

Japanese facial massage is an advanced modality of massage that treats surface and deep facial tissues, *tsubo*, and meridians with highly refined hand techniques in accordance with traditional Japanese medical theory.

If you are used to giving full-body massages, you will notice a difference in the applications of Japanese facial massage. The application of facial massage is similar to Japanese foot massage—it is a more difficult and advanced form than regular full-body massage. Full-body massage is primarily applied with the hands (rather than fingers), and the force of the massage comes from broad movements of the shoulder, elbow, and wrist. Japanese facial massage involves techniques, the majority of which use finger movements and manipulations within the hands, and requires precise finger manipulation. Some of the important techniques require the practitioner to coordinate the left and right hands to a degree uncommon in other modalities. Several techniques require the left and right hands to apply different applications simultaneously.

Often it is difficult for the beginning practitioner to control the non-dominant hand and finger movements to the degree necessary for good facial massage. It is important to practice until both the right and left hand and fingers move smoothly and comfortably. The best way to do this is to learn each technique thoroughly with your dominant hand, and then let this hand teach your non-dominant hand to do the stroke. If your hands are unbalanced in the application, and if you are uncomfortable with these techniques, the client will sense this and will not be able to relax properly. Practice until you are comfortable with the strokes.

How Japanese Facial Massage Differs From Western Facial Massage

Although my foundation has been in Japanese medicine and massage, I have studied and practiced Western facial-massage techniques. I recognize the value of these Western modalities, and I appreciate the diligence that students are putting into the study of these techniques. But I do know that there are many common conditions that Western facial-massage techniques cannot address— conditions that Japanese methods treat routinely with tremendous result. The two modalities are similar only to a certain point. It must be remembered that, in Japan, massage is and has been a legitimate branch of medicine used in the treatment of disease as well as in the therapeutic treatment of the facial tissues.

There are distinct differences between Japanese and Western facial massages. As I explained in the previous chapter, the conceptual foundation of health and medicine is completely different in Japan. Additionally, there are also many technical differences in hand and finger applications.

The greatest difference between the two approaches is the rich knowledge of *ki* flow in the Japanese tradition. Although both Japanese and Western modalities focus on the condition of the skin and muscles, the Japanese approach begins with attention to the basic energetic health of the body and tissues. Knowledge of the *ki* flow in the face and the ability to balance this flow of the internal organs and consequently balance emotional conditions are very important—and unique—characteristics of Japanese facial massage.

Japanese facial massage utilizes a much larger and more varied repertoire of techniques than Western massage. The Western massage repertoire uses many techniques similar to Japanese techniques, but the Japanese repertoire has a far greater range and much more refined application of such techniques.

The core of Western facial-massage technique is a smooth light stroking of the surface tissues. Japanese facial massage is based on percussive techniques and combines these with a deep-kneading technique to work the musculature underneath the surface tissues. Japanese massage also uses a variety of surface strokes.

Another important difference between the two is that Japanese facial massage uses much deeper pressure than Western facial massage. To reach the deeper musculature, a variety of percussive and kneading techniques are combined and a range of pressure applied to areas that are treated lightly in Western facial massage. However, these deep routines require direct supervision and are therefore not introduced in this popular edition of the Japanese facial-massage manual. Japanese massage has a greater range of therapeutic applications; during a single massage the practitioner utilizes extremely light stroking to move the lymphatic fluid and deep pressure to loosen the tight facial muscles. This dynamic range of Japanese facial- massage techniques allows the practitioner to give a much more effective treatment than the Western modalities allow.

In addition to the moisturizing and cleansing stages that Western massage modalities use, Japanese facial massage adds a third stage, called an energizing stage, which adds tremendous benefit to the entire facial massage, producing the effect of a natural face-lift without needing to insert the needles as used in acupuncture (and without, of course, the side effects of a surgical procedure!).

The energizing stage works directly with *ki*—the very life force of the human body—stimulating important *tsubo* (acupoints/acupuncture points) and stroking certain meridians in the face to enhance the *ki* flow of the face and the corresponding organs to balance the physical body. According to Japanese medical tradition and clinical experience, the condition of the physical body and the emotional condition reflect one another, and both hinge on the state of *ki* flow. Balancing the *ki* flow brings the body and emotions into balance simultaneously.

Japanese facial massages utilize the concept of Japanese facial diagnosis, meridians (*keiraku*), and *tsubo* to help balance the client's emotions. Japanese facial massage uses facial diagnosis methods to identify each client's internal organ imbalances.

Practitioners of traditional Japanese medicine observe facial skin conditions to determine a person's health, both physical and psychological. The Japanese concept holds that the face reflects the condition of the entire body; in treating facial conditions at the professional level, it is essential to understand the condition of the entire body. The treatment proceeds holistically. Poor facial tone can come from factors such as poor diet, stress, or lifestyle change, and you must determine the particular cause of a client's poor health to treat effectively.

Japanese facial massage generally begins with an effective neck massage to improve blood flow to the face. Proper blood flow is essential for the face to repair damaged tissues, flush toxins, and to supply facial tissues with oxygen and other nutrients. Neck massage also provides a relaxing introduction to the facial therapy: in general, people carry such a concentrated degree of tension in the neck muscles that initial attention to this area encourages immediate relaxation.

When we give a Japanese facial massage, we dislodge toxins that rise to the skin surface from various facial tissues. It is important to flush these toxins into the lymphatic system so they can be expelled naturally. To do this, we apply very light strokes, called finishing touch strokes, which drain toxins from the face.

Wrinkles are not easy to treat by conventional therapeutic measures, such as steam baths, mud masks, and creams. These methods treat only the skin surface and the superficial layers just beneath the surface. Wrinkles are a product of gradual malnourishment of the skin cells and must be treated with deeper therapy. Japanese facial massage stimulates the facial nerves which reach the skin cells, improving the flow of blood, the distribution of nutrients, and the removal of toxins and dead skin cells. This allows the skin to rebuild itself. It is the most effective natural treatment for wrinkles and the best prevention against them.

The face is a complex network of muscles which are used constantly. Smiling, chewing, laughing, speaking, sneezing, and yawning all cause facial muscles to contract. As a result, the facial muscles are in almost constant use and begin to collect tension. Eventually, this causes constriction of muscle tissues and a decrease in circulation to the surface tissues. When blood is unable to circulate properly through these tissues, the facial tissue near the surface begins to decay. The face becomes stiff, and the tissue begins to lose its natural elasticity: it is being choked and suffocated to death.

Japanese facial massage uses very small yet deep muscle-manipulation techniques to release over-contracted muscular tissue. This unblocks the restriction of blood flow and allows fresh blood to circulate to enter the surface of the face, giving oxygen and nutrition to the skin cells. Only when this circulation is unimpeded can skin cells repair and rejuvenate themselves.

Japanese facial massage is capable of treating a full range of facial problems, from surface conditions such as dry and oily skin, acne, wrinkles, age spots, and poor facial tone, to more difficult conditions such as migraines, headaches, and temporo-mandibular joint (TMJ) disorders. Japanese facial massage is not merely versatile, it is also extremely effective; there is virtually no other modality that achieves the therapeutic standards of properly applied Japanese facial massage.

As I mentioned earlier, Japanese facial massage is a subject which goes beyond simply massaging the face. It is an art for understanding each individual's health condition, in the traditional paradigm of physical, psychological, and spiritual balance. As it is a traditional art, it is not easily mastered. One can master the techniques themselves in a relatively short period of time. But one comes to the essence of Japanese facial massage only after many years of study, and it takes a lifetime to combine all the elements masterfully in a style of one's own.

Chapter Four

ANATOMY OF THE FACE

P erforming Japanese facial massage does not require knowledge or experience of other styles of massage, nor is it necessary to have a complete understanding of the anatomy or physiology of the face to give a good facial massage. Of course, this information is helpful and will be introduced as necessary. In the East, we have been giving facial massage for centuries, yet have only understood the anatomy and physiology of the human body for less than 200 years. In massage therapy, it is more important to understand anatomy with one's hands than to possess a complete academic knowledge of it. The study of technical anatomy is helpful, however, and you may find that it complements your massage practice.

Anatomical language is used to communicate between therapists to minimize confusion and indicate precise locations. For example, the area just below the eye can be understood to be in a different location depending on whether the person is standing and facing forward or lying down and facing forward. This chapter explains basic terminology to reduce misunderstandings during explanations of the techniques. This book (the popular edition) has eliminated most of the anatomical terminology and has substituted simpler phrases, keeping necessary terminology in parentheses.

The diagrams in this chapter show the basic structure of the bones and muscles of the face. The only information that will be crucial for you to use this book are the locations of the zygomatic bones and arches. These should be very easy to memorize. As everyone's facial contour is unique, the exact skeletal and muscular structures of individual faces are slightly different, so these diagrams provide general guidelines to work from and the practitioner must adjust accordingly.

Inner Hand and Outer Hand

In this book, you will occasionally see the terms "inner hand" and "outer hand" used only when the face is in the tilted position. The inner hand is the hand which is nearest to the center of the client's face. I use the term "inner thumb," or "inner fingers," and "outer thumb," or "outer fingers." These refer to the thumb or fingers of the inner hand or the thumb or fingers of the outer hand.

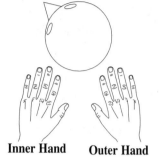

Inner Hand   Outer Hand

For the sake of consistency, all examples shown in this book are demonstrated and explained on the client's right side of the face. I have arranged the text this way because most people find it easier to learn on the right side of the face. To work on the left side of the face, reverse the directions and hand positions. Each example should be performed on both sides of the face. Be sure to practice on the both the right and left sides of the face until you are comfortable with each. In an actual facial massage, it is common to completely work on one side of the face before working on the other.

Anterior/Posterior

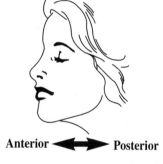

Anterior ◄——► Posterior

Anterior refers to the direction toward the front of the body, or it references the front of another identifying feature on the body. Posterior is the opposite direction, referring to the direction toward the back of the body. With the face viewed from the side, if a person moves the finger from the ear to the nose, he or she has has moved anteriorly; the nose is anterior to the ear. If the person move the finger from the ear to the back of the head (to the occiput, for example), he or she has moved posteriorly; the back of the head is posterior to the ear.

Superior/Inferior

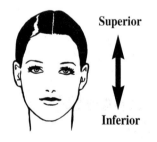

Superior

Inferior

Superior refers to the direction toward the top of the head, and inferior refers to the direction toward the feet. Moving the finger from the ear to the top of the head is moving superiorly—the top of the head is superior to the ear. Moving the finger from the ear to the neck is moving inferiorly—the neck is inferior to the ear.

Medial/Lateral

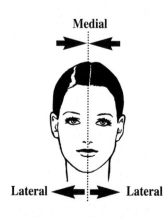

Medial

Lateral ◄——► Lateral

Medial refers toward the center (median) line of the face or a motion toward the center. Lateral refers moving from the center line of the face or in a direction away from the center. Moving a finger from one ear to the nose is a medial movement—the nose is medial to the ear. Moving the finger from the nose to the ear is a lateral movement—the ear is lateral to the nose. This same movement can be described in terms of its movement anteriorly or posteriorly, as above.

Specific Regions of the Face

These are brief definitions of terms used to describe different regions of the face. Each example describes a slightly different and more specific area of the face to avoid confusion.

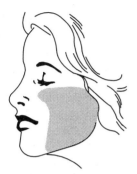

Cheek Region

The large fleshy portion of skin between the eye, nose, ear, and jaw.

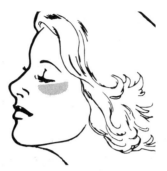

Below the Eye

The area just inferior to the eye, over the upper edge of the zygomatic bone.

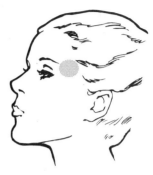

Temporal Region

The area between the eyebrow and hairline, just posterior to the lateral edge of eyebrow.

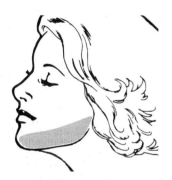

Along the Jaw

The skin area that runs along the jaw bone, below the cheek and between the chin and the ear.

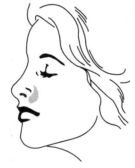

Side of Nose

The region around the crease, just lateral to the lower portion of the nose (nare).

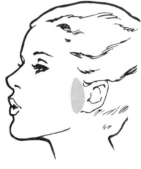

In front of the Ear

The region just anterior to the attachment of the ear.

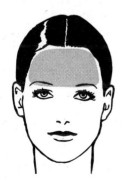

Forehead

The entire region between the hairline and the eyebrows.

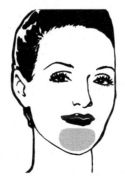

Chin

The area inferior to the lower lip and superior to the jaw line.

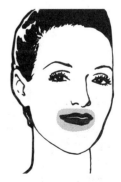

Around the Mouth

The area that immediately surrounds the lips and that moves with the mouth.

Bones of the Face

The skull and face are comprised of several bones which are not flexible. Basically, the head has two main bones: the skull and jawbone, and the jawbone, while attached to the skull, is quite mobile.

It is not necessary to know the names of the bones which comprise the skull to make use of this book. It is helpful become familiar with the location of the zygomatic bone, commonly called the cheekbone.

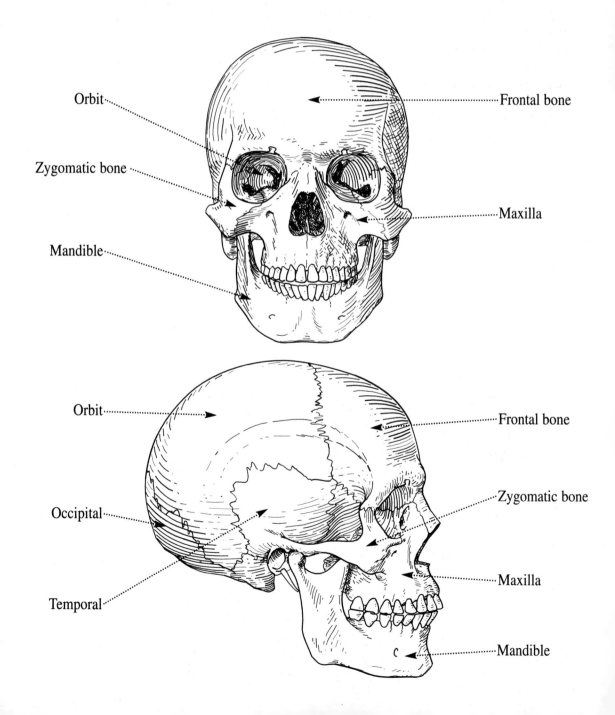

Orbit — Frontal bone

Zygomatic bone

Maxilla

Mandible

Orbit — Frontal bone

Zygomatic bone

Occipital

Maxilla

Temporal

Mandible

Muscles of the Face

The muscles of the face are complex. Because the face performs a number of varied and separate movements to create expressions and show emotions and along with the muscle support necessary for ingesting and chewing food, many muscles are required to support and execute these movements.

It is not essential to memorize the name for every single muscle of the face. It is more important to have a general idea of where the muscles are located, how big they are, and in which direction they are running. The majority of the muscles is located around the eyes and around the mouth. The jaw muscle is one of the strongest muscles in the entire body, as well as one of the first muscles in the body to develop due to its critical role in the proper ingestion of food for the body's survival. The major muscles are shown here, but for a more detailed understanding of the anatomy of the face, please refer to a good anatomy or cadaver reference book.

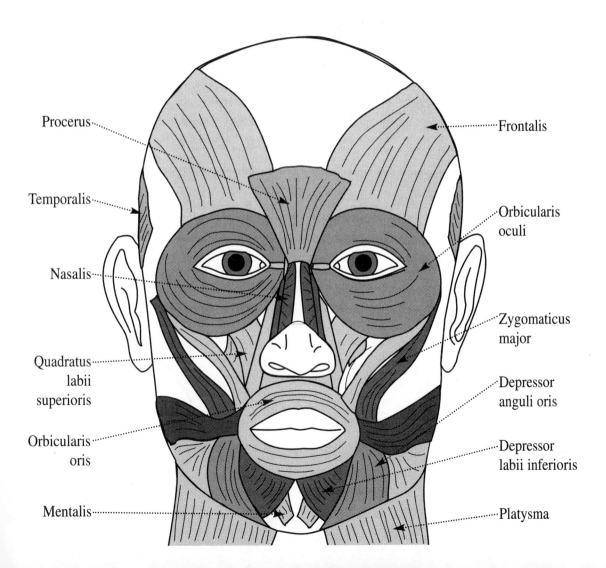

Chapter Five

THE APPLICATION OF

JAPANESE FACIAL MASSAGE

In this chapter, I explain the basics for the application of Japanese facial massage, including preparatory steps (how to get the client set up on a table or floor mat) and precautions to help you better perform Japanese facial massage. I also provide ideas for the protection and maintenance of your hands during application that are useful for practitioners of any modality of massage and bodywork. This chapter provides answers to the most common questions about the application of Japanese facial massage.

Chapter 6 explains the basic hand-application techniques used in Japanese facial massage. It is best to have a clear understanding of the differing characteristics of each individual hand-application technique before attempting to perform Japanese facial massage. Chapters 7 through 10 introduce appropriate techniques for specific regions of the neck and face. These examples help you to understand how to combine basic techniques when working on particular regions. For example, one particular technique may work well along the jaw, but that same technique may not be appropriate for other areas of the face. These differences must be mastered to determine which technique are the the most effective for a particular condition.

Whether you are a beginner or are already proficient in other forms of massage, you should begin practicing massage on a partner who can provide constructive feedback. It is important to remember that levels of sensitivity differ between individuals. Learn from your partner's feedback and adjust your techniques appropriately.

Understanding basic procedures and guidelines are the first steps in learning to perform Japanese facial massage. You will learn fifty-five different techniques, and you must practice each of them thoroughly before attempting a complete facial massage. To follow are a few general tips that will help you learn the application of a basic facial massage.

Tips for Getting Started

Japanese facial massage can be performed on the floor with a mat, in a reclining chair, or on a massage table. If using a massage table, you should adjust it properly. Additionally, the environment should be quiet, properly lit, and temperate. You can also add some soft, relaxing music.

Use your dominant hand when learning a new technique. If you are right-handed, practice the technique on the right side of the client's face. All examples in Chapters 7 through 10 are explained on the right side of the client's face, neck, or head. Once you become comfortable with the application of a technique using your dominant hand, reverse the hand placements and practice on the other side of the face. For the majority of the techniques, keep your shoulders down, elbows dropped, and wrists relaxed.

How to Practice Japanese Facial Massage

Before applying the techniques on a client or friend, try them on yourself if possible (some techniques may be difficult to apply). This should be done to determine how much pressure should be applied and to understand the correct way of performing the movement. In many of these techniques, a detail such as the angle of your fingers can either make the technique feel enjoyable or uncomfortable. Of course, individuals have different levels of comfort with regard to degree of pressure and touch, so it is important to understand the proper application of the techniques and amount of pressure to apply. The facial massage should not be applied too lightly as there will be no therapeutic benefits; however, working too deeply can cause stress and discomfort to the facial skin and eliminate the therapeutic effects.

Each massage technique can be applied with different levels of pressure, and various parts of the body can absorb different amounts of pressure. Experience will inform you as to how much pressure should be applied where and when. As you begin working with people, be sure to communicate verbally. It is appropriate to ask them, "Is this comfortable?" or "Is this too much or too light pressure?". Developing rapport with your client and soliciting feedback helps you gain a sense of the appropriate level of pressure to use with each client.

Japanese Face Massage: Before and After

It is helpful to warm the face with a moist heating pad or towel before and after the facial massage. The application of heat increases circulation, rid the face of toxins, and help your client relax. The temperature must be warm but not too hot. Although it is preferable to use a heating device (such as a towel warmer), heating a wet towel in a crock pot may be substituted. Do not use an electric heating pad or blanket.

It is best if the client does not wear make-up before the facial massage, and if the client arrives for the appointment with make-up on, it must be removed. In Japan, alcohol (such as *sake*, which is rice wine, or *sho chu*, which is Japanese vodka) was traditionally used to remove make-up and clean the face, but it tends to be harsh on the skin. I recommend finding a gentle astringent or toner to remove the make-up. If possible, use the toner instead of astringent, as toner does not contain alcohol and is more gentle on the skin. During make-up removal, do not use paper tissues. Facial-tissue paper is essentially a wood product. The tissue paper contains fine slivers of wood and can scratch the face at a microscopic level. It is best to use cotton balls, pads, or products made of 100% cotton, because they are much softer and there is less chance of scratching the facial skin. Avoid blended-cotton products, such as 50% polyester/cotton blends, because they can also scratch the face. After the massage, wipe the face with a dry towel, or steam the face with a warm wet towel and wipe it afterward. Warming the face for one to two minutes is sufficient. Do not allow the towel to become chilled, as cold decreases circulation in the face and nullifies the benefits of a facial massage.

After the treatment, have the client drink water to help flush toxins from the body. It is important that your client drink about two cups of pure water, ideally warm or lukewarm. Warmer water is preferred because cold water chills the internal organs and decreases circulation. Tea, coffee, soda, or even juices are not suitable substitutes. If your client does not drink enough water, these toxins stay in the bloodstream, and the effects of the massage will be lessened. If your client has heart, liver, or kidney disease, the amount should be reduced to about three-quarters of a cup.

Applications for Clients with Injuries or Surgery

You can still perform facial massage on a client who has had recent surgery or an injury to the face or neck, as long as it has healed properly and there are no open wounds. Applying a neck and facial massage may require extra caution. For neck massage, use much lighter pressure, especially for the first five examples discussed in this book. It is best to avoid massage following facial plastic/reconstructive surgery; consult with the client's physician about readiness. Regardless, always avoid working directly on bruises, stitches, or broken skin.

Japanese Facial Massage and Lubrication

In Japan, many things are used as traditional ingredients in making cosmetics. Some of these items include the leaves, barks, and roots of trees; oils from various plants; and fruits, vegetables (such as cucumbers), and grains. There are wonderful effects from using fresh and natural ingredients, but they can be very inconvenient to prepare for use with just a few massages per day.

Different products are required for different conditions, and it becomes impossible to have that amount of fresh produce on hand daily. It also takes time to prepare many of the items (for example, there are many beans that need to be soaked, cooked, and chilled overnight before use). Also, preparations using fresh vegetables last only a few days at most. In general practice, it is easier to rely on commercial products, and you can still find natural consumer products that work well for you and your client.

There are two basic categories of facial products that you must have: a cleanser and a moisturizer. Cleanser is used during the first stage of the facial massage. The main focus of the cleanser is to remove excess oil and dirt from the face. I highly recommend using a water-based cleanser rather than an oil-based one. Moisturizer is used during the moisturizing, energizing, and finishing-touch stages.

Also, toner and masks are commonly used during modern Japanese facial massage. The purpose of toner is to remove make-up or excess cleansers or moisturizers and to balance the pH of the skin during facial massage. Masks restore moisture, vitamins, and minerals to the skin, rejuvenating the condition of the skin .

Generally, facial products sold in department stores are not made for use in facial massage. There are a few products (generally Japanese and French) that are made for facial massage, and are labeled as a facial-massage cream or a facial-massage moisturizer. While you can use a generic body-massage oil for the moisturizing stage, I do not recommend it. Petroleum products and by-products are commonly known to be improper for use on the face because they clog the pores. Their use on the face has been controversial. Also, it is best to avoid artificial coloring in moisturizers and cleansers. If you are working professionally, you should use facial products from one of the many excellent professional cosmetic product lines.

Each person's face has different sensitivities and needs. If you work on a number of people, you will find that there are no products that can be used universally on every face without eventually creating problems. You must have different products for different facial conditions, such as separate products for either an oily or dry face.

Natural or hypoallergenic products do not guarantee that your client won't have an allergic reaction to the product. Allergies are very pervasive, and it is impossible to predict what could trigger a reaction in your client. Always ask your client to confirm which products are preferable for use or if there is any history of allergic reactions to particular skin products. Avoid products with multiple ingredients or have strong fragrances that can cause skin irritations. You should always be equipped with fragrance-free cleanser and moisturizer. Also, many people are allergic to the individual ingredients in some products. If a reaction is going to occur, it usually happen quite quickly. Immediately remove the product if it irritates or gives any sensation to the facial skin.

The quality of the cleanser and moisturizer is important, but the texture is a key factor. Both cleanser and moisturizer must have textures that are sufficiently lubricating for a smooth massage. It is critical to have the correct texture in the cleanser first rather than the moisturizer, because in Japanese facial massage, more time is spent on the cleansing stage. Even some expensive organic products are too stiff or too liquid for use in massage. If the product is too stiff, it pulls the skin. If it's too liquid, it slips too much.

Besides the texture, it is also important that the moisturizer remain moist for the somewhat extended time frame that is required in working on the face. It should not be so dry that you must keep adding more moisturizer.

When you are not using the facial products, it is best to store them in the refrigerator after opening, as it can increase the life of the product. Be sure to bring facial products to room temperature prior to use. Every product has its own shelf life: do not use a product that is outdated. If a product starts to show a color or texture change, regardless of how expensive it is, throw it out and replace it with a new one. If a product comes in a jar, remove the amount needed for your massage with a knife or spoon. Do not use your fingers to remove creams or oils from a jar, as you can easily contaminate the container and the product left within it.

You must carefully examine the condition of each of your client's faces and choose the proper product for the best results. The amount of product, the amount of pressure used with the technique, and the duration and frequency of treatment are factors which must be balanced and carefully adjusted to suit each individual's conditions.

Duration and Frequency of Treatments

As I explained earlier, Japanese facial massage is done in three stages—cleansing, moisturizing, and energizing. The duration of Japanese facial massage (including neck and scalp massage) is about fifteen to twenty-five minutes. It can be performed by applying the facial massage alone or as part of an entire body massage. The length of the massage depends upon how much time is available, as well as the age, personal needs, and facial conditions of your client.

The frequency of Japanese facial massage is very important. Develop a regular schedule with your client, such as once a week or every ten days. I do not recommend receiving facial massage more than once a week. Overstimulation can create negative effects. It is much more effective for the client to receive Japanese facial massage on a regular basis than it is to receive many sessions in a short period of time and then skip several months.

Generally, between ten to twenty minutes is a comfortable amount of time for a Japanese facial massage. A facial massage should not take any more than twenty-five minutes. Again, overstimulation of the face can cause negative results, such as creating dark spots on the skin. Facial massage of more than thirty minutes drains the therapist and overworks the client. If you are not able to complete a massage in one session, another visit should be arranged.

Combining Japanese Facial Massage with Other Massage

The Japanese facial massage can be easily incorporated into a full anma, shiatsu, or Western massage routine. You can also incorporate these Japanese facial-massage techniques into other styles of facial massage or use it to enhance the techniques of cosmetologists or estheticians.

Japanese facial massage can be combined with any style of massage during any part of the massage routine. It works best when the client is most calm and relaxed. When combining Japanese facial massage with other practices, a ten-to fifteen-minute application is usually sufficient. Remember: always massage the face **before** massaging the feet.

If you are giving a facial massage alone as a professional service, some states require special licensing, such as cosmetology or esthetology licenses. If you are applying a facial massage as part of a full-body massage or combined with other massage and bodywork, it generally requires only a massage-therapy license or certification.

Before Applying Japanese Facial Massage

I recommend following these simple guidelines before applying a facial massage:

1. To eliminate bacterial infections, keep your fingernails short.
2. Keep your hands clean. Wash them with antibacterial soap immediately prior to each massage session.
3. Remove your watch when applying a massage so that tendons in the wrist are not restricted. Also remove all rings and jewelry from your hands and wrists.
4. Warm up, stretch, and massage your fingers, hands and arms.
5. Inquire if your client has had any injuries, surgery, and/or health problems, especially on the neck.
6. Inquire if your client has any history of allergic reactions or problems with oils or other skin products.
7. Inquire if your client has any communicable diseases which you should be aware of, such as flu or tuberculosis.
8. Relax the client and yourself.
9. Your hands should be warm for initial contact.

Minor adjustments may be required when applying Japanese facial massage on infants, the elderly, or persons with injuries or illnesses. Some techniques may require modifications to fit the smaller faces of infants or children.

Your client should:

1. Clean the face thoroughly and remove make-up.
2. Remove all facial, neck, and ear jewelry.
3. Remove glasses or contact lenses.
4. Wear comfortable clothes so that the neck is easily accessible.
5. Avoid being extremely hungry or full during a treatment.
6. Drink water after the massage.

Do not apply Japanese facial massage if the client suffers from:

1. A fever.
2. A contagious illness.
3. Has had recent surgery, especially on the neck or face.
4. Skin infections, rashes, or a severe break-out of the skin.

Remember that you have the right to refuse any client a massage if you suspect a condition which could be contagious, such as open sores on the face. Another option is to use non-latex surgical gloves, since most of the techniques can be performed using gloves. Regardless, it is always best to have surgical gloves on hand whenever you perform massage. Always wash with antibacterial soap before and immediately after treatment to reduce the risk of infections. Have your client consult a doctor if you or the client are in doubt about a medical condition.

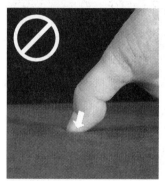

Rotating with the thumb joint

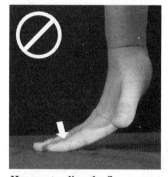

Pressure with a bent thumb

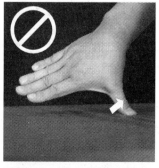

Hyperextending the fingers

Hyperextending the thumb

Using and Developing the Thumb

Japanese facial massage contains much more finger manipulation than hand manipulation. This can exhaust the finger muscles or overwork the thumb. For the intensive techniques of Japanese facial massage, it is important to develop strength in your fingers, thumbs, and especially the muscles which support the thumbs. If you are not accustomed to using your thumb muscles, they will tire quickly and easily. To give the thumb recovery time during treatment, it helps to alternate techniques which do and do not use the thumb with applications. Development of these muscles is one of the essential requirements for mastering Japanese facial massage. The best method for developing the thumb is to perform facial massage often.

Some Techniques to Avoid

Many massage therapists complain of problems in the hands or fingers. The practitioner should always properly warm up the hands before working on a client. Stretch and massage your hands before and after applying Japanese facial massage to keep them in the best possible working condition.

You should not have any stress, pain, or overstretched feelings in your hands, fingers, wrists, elbows, or shoulders while performing a massage. These sensations indicate incorrect applications or positioning. You must check your hand application and readjust to find the correct, comfortable position. Protecting yourself is the first priority. An injury built up over time can ruin a therapist's hands (and the business practice as well). The following are some common mistakes made in applications and how to correct them.

1) Do not rotate with your thumb while applying heavy pressure (rotation from the metacarpals). This causes significant wear on the thumb joints and cartilage. Instead, apply pressure with the thumb and use the rest of your hand for stability. Rotate by using the whole hand from the shoulder or from the elbow.

2) Do not apply pressure with a bent thumb. Applying pressure when bending your thumb puts pressure on the joint instead of on the client. Keep the thumb straight and apply pressure perpendicularly to reduce stress and prevent premature wear on the joints.

3) Do not overextend the fingers (bend backward) to apply pressure. Instead, support the fingers by slightly rotating your wrist and placing adjacent fingers behind or alongside of each other.

4) Do not stroke or apply pressure with the side of the thumb or allow it to hyperextend as you stroke, as this creates stress to the carpometacarpal and metacarpophalangeal joints. Change the angle of the thumb to push into the stroke with the hand.

Hand-Maintenance Method:

As a massage therapist, especially at the professional level, it is important that you properly maintain your hands. Many hand problems can be prevented, reduced, or eliminated by performing a daily maintenance massage on your own hands and forearms. When working for several hours at a time, it is essential that you massage and stretch your hands frequently. This is especially important when you feel tightness in your forearms and hands, a condition which often occurs in the morning after a day of performing massage.

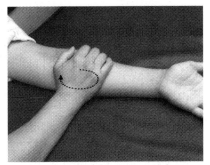

Palm rotation on the forearm

You must properly warm and loosen the muscles before performing a massage. Spend about five minutes stretching and massaging your fingers, hands, wrists, arms, and shoulders before and after each massage. I teach my students a routine of twenty-five techniques to maintain the hands. Here are four of the most important techniques.

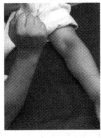
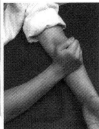

1. Palm Rotation on the Forearm
Place your arm on the massage table with the palm facing up. Grasp the inner (medial) edge of the forearm with the palm of your other hand. Apply pressure onto your forearm and rotate, using your entire shoulder and arm. Continue applying rotation to the entire forearm until it is warm.

Percussion on the forearm

2. Percussion on the Forearm
Position your arm as you did in the previous technique. Make a loose fist with your other hand. Strike your forearm with the loose fist, keeping your wrist loose. You can strike with the front of your fist, the side of your wrist, or the back of your hand. Again, cover your entire forearm.

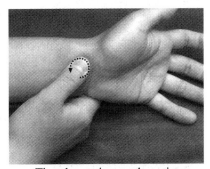

Thumb rotation on the wrist

3. Thumb Rotation on the Wrist
Place your thumb on the inner side of the wrist, just below the other thumb, and wrap the fingers around behind the wrist for support. Apply rotation by using your entire hand (not just the thumb). Move the thumb across the middle of the wrist, working your way to the inner side of the hand (hypothenar side) and repeat the rotation. Repeat the whole sequence on the other side of the wrist.

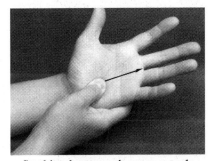

Stroking between the metacarpals

4. Stroking Between the Metacarpals
Place your thumb on the heel of your hand, wrapping the fingers around behind the hand for support. Use the thumb to stroke slowly between the metacarpal bones. Begin just above the wrist and end between the base of each finger. Work between all of the metacarpals (including between the thumb and index finger). Repeat the stroking on the other side of the hand. Lubrication can be used if needed.

> For further information:
> ***Hand Maintenance Guide***
> ***for Massage Therapists***
> Kotobuki Publications
> see the back of this book
> for details.

Client Positioning for Japanese Facial Massage

Japanese facial massage is generally applied with the client lying on the back (supine position). It is extremely rare to apply in other positions, such as on the side or in a sitting position.

There are a variety of ways to set up for Japanese facial massage. A massage or salon table is often used, but not everyone has a table and some people may prefer to work on the floor. A reclining chair can be used. Whichever arrangement you choose, it is important that you position yourself comfortably in relation to the client's face and neck, so that it is easier for you to apply the facial massage and better minimize the stress to your body. Make sure that your client is positioned comfortably as well.

Japanese facial massage can be applied on a regular massage table, which should be sturdy and not squeak. The fabric should be water- and oil-resistant for easy cleaning and sanitizing between massages. The massage table should be adjusted to the easiest position for the therapist to work from: not too high or too low. It is important to adjust the height of the massage table rather than have the therapist adjust to an uncomfortable position.

Regardless of whether you are working on a massage table or on the floor, there should be a sheet or cover between the client and the surface. Using a twin-sized sheet under the client works well for most tables. If you are working on a sofa or reclining chair, you should place a large towel under the head to protect the fabric from lubricant. The rest of the client's body should be covered for warmth. Sheets and towels must be changed between each massage.

A small pillow or bolster can be placed under the client's knee for comfort. A peaceful and quiet environment can enhance the massage as well. It is best to apply the massage in a warm and quiet room. Interruptions and noises, such as phone calls, should be minimized. Soft, soothing music can also be added for relaxation.

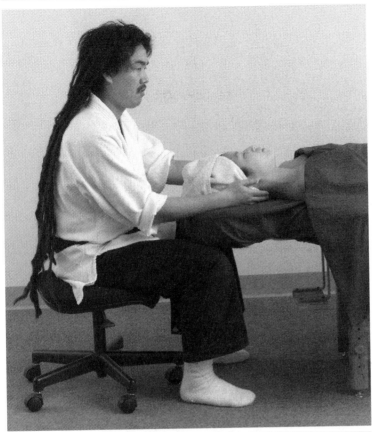

Japanese facial massage is most often performed on a massage table but can also be performed on the floor.

Massage-Table Settings for Japanese Facial Massage

Japanese facial-massage techniques work well when performed on a massage table set at a regular height. If you are using a salon-style table, the angle of the upper body should be as low as possible to minimize stress to the wrist and shoulder of the person applying the massage. A massage table should not be set too high or too low. Generally, I do not place a pillow under the client's head. Sit on a chair at the head of the table and adjust the height so that the face is level with your chest.

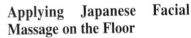

Applying Japanese Facial Massage on the Floor

Since all Japanese massage is traditionally performed on the floor, the techniques work well without the use of a massage table. If you are combining Japanese facial massage with anma, shiatsu, or other bodywork, you will find they compliment each other.

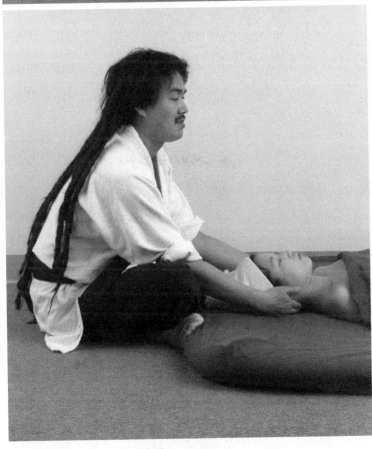

You can have your client lay on a thin futon, pad, or carpeted floor for comfort. You can add a small pillow under the client's head or a larger pillow to slightly raise the entire upper body, making it easier for the therapist. Many westerners are not accustomed to kneeling for long periods of time. You can sit on a pillow or cushion for comfort.

Chapter Six

THE BASIC TECHNIQUES OF JAPANESE FACIAL MASSAGE

In this chapter, I introduce the hand-manipulation techniques of Japanese facial massage. The majority of Japanese facial-massage techniques originate from anma and have been modified over a period of time to work specifically on the face.

The many techniques of Japanese facial massage are divided into categories. Each category has its own unique character and purpose that are explained in this chapter. It is important to have a clear understanding of the differences between the characteristics of each category of techniques. Memorizing these categories makes it much easier for you to differentiate between the dozens of techniques as you learn them.

Chapters 7 through 10 provide examples of massage techniques to show how each is performed. To effectively learn Japanese facial massage, you must first learn each example of the technique individually. Initially this may seem very fragmented, but it is very important to understand the qualities and purpose of each technique before stringing them together. Later in your training, you will learn to combine them fluently to develop a smooth, coordinated massage.

For those familiar with anma, I have included Japanese terminology for easy reference. It is not necessary to memorize these words in order to practice Japanese facial massage, nor is an understanding of Japanese language or culture needed to understand the techniques.

Japanese Facial-Massage Application Techniques

Japanese facial-massage application techniques are mainly derived from anma. Anma is constructed of seven foundational categories of techniques:

1. *kei satsu ho*	light-stroking techniques
2. *ju netsu ho*	kneading techniques
3. *shin sen ho*	vibrating techniques
4. *ap paku ho*	pressure techniques
5. *ko da ho*	percussion techniques
6. *kyoku te ho*	special percussion techniques
7. *un do ho*	movement and stretching techniques

The kneading techniques (*ju netsu ho*) are the primary techniques used in anma. In Japanese facial massage, the stroking techniques (*kei satsu ho*) and special percussion techniques (*kyoku te ho*) are the foundational techniques. The kneading techniques (*ju netsu ho*), the pressure techniques (*ap paku ho*), and the stretching techniques (*un do ho*) are used together to enhance the effects of the massage.

Anma also has supplemental techniques which are less often used:

8. *kyo satsu ho*	stroking/rotating with heavy pressure
9. *ha aku ho*	gripping and squeezing techniques
10. *ken biki ho*	pulling and traction techniques
11. *shin kin ho*	stretching the muscles or fascia

I also briefly introduce five shiatsu techniques in this chapter, although they are used infrequently. Because shiatsu grew out of anma, the nature of the techniques is very similar. Understanding anma techniques is sufficient to give Japanese facial massage. Each technique is unique in character and offers different effects. Combining techniques offers better and faster results than simply performing one technique repeatedly. As you progress in your practice of massage, you will develop a sense of how to combine techniques efficiently to offer the correct technique in the appropriate situation. As you begin combining techniques, select a few and try to alternate between them smoothly. You will eventually learn to make only marginal changes in the amount of force and speed used in each technique.

Another reason for combining techniques is that different techniques require the use of different muscles in your hand. By frequently alternating between techniques, you can avoid over-exerting one particular part of the hand. Also, the muscles that are used for movement during application are less likely to tire.

For further information about the application of Japanese Massage techniques, refer to the book:

ANMA: The Art of Japanese Massage

See back of this book for details.

How to Understand the Japanese Characters of Techniques

Throughout this book I have included the Japanese names of the hand-manipulation techniques for each example. Although it is not necessary to memorize all of these names, you should memorize at least the names of the basic techniques and pressure points if you are serious about your Japanese facial-massage practice. To advance in the study of any traditional Japanese medicine, it is important for Westerners to understand the rudiments of the native language. It has been my experience that most of my students enjoy learning and understanding the names and technical language of Japanese facial massage, anma, and shiatsu.

Below is an example which shows how common Japanese facial-massage and anma techniques are named in Japanese.

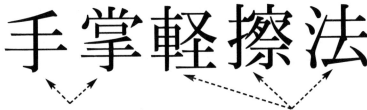

The first two (sometimes three) characters show which part of the hand the massage is applied with. In this case, *shu sho* indicates the entire palm.

The next three characters explain which technique is being applied. The last character is always "*ho*," which means "technique". This example shows *kei satsu ho*, a light stroking technique.

This set of characters means—"a light stroking technique applied with the entire palm." Below are some examples of the first two or three characters that indicate which part of the hand is used to apply the appropriate technique.

手掌 ***shu sho***

Shu sho means "entire palm of the hand." Generally, it includes the insides of the fingers and the sides of the thumbs.

拇指 ***bo shi***

Bo means "mother" and *shi* means "finger." Together, they have come to mean thumb. *Bo shi* usually refers to the inside of the thumb.

拇指頭 ***bo shi to***

Bo shi means "thumb" and *to* means the "tip" or "head," so *bo shi to* is the tip of thumb.

二指 ***ni shi***

Ni shi means "the flat parts of two fingers." Normally, *ni shi* refers to the index and middle fingers, but it can also refer to other combinations of two fingers

四指頭 ***shi shi to***

Shi shi means "four fingers" and *to* means "tip" or "head," so *shi shi to* means "the tips of the four fingers."

手拳 ***shu ken***

Shu ken means "hand-staff," and includes the top of the middle phalanges, the distal phalanges, or the top of the metacarpophalangeal and interphalangeal joints.

拇指球 ***bo shi kyu***

Bo shi means "thumb" and *kyu* means "ball," so this is the thenar (radial-carpal ball) region of the inner hand.

小指球 ***ko shi kyu***

Ko shi means "pinky" and *kyu* means "ball," so this is the hypothenar region of the palmer hand (ulnar-carpal ball).

手根 ***shu kon***

Shu kon refers to the region directly over the carpal bones which form the heel of the hand.

1. Light-Stroking Technique—*Kei Satsu Ho*

軽擦法

Kei satsu ho

按撫法

(Also known as *an bu ho*)

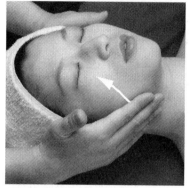

Stroking with four fingers

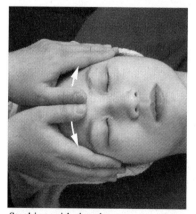

Stroking with thumbs

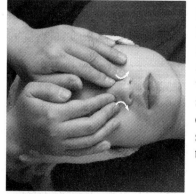

Stroking with two fingers

Light-stroking technique, or *kei satsu ho*, is performed by sliding over the surface with either up-and-down or circular motions. This is one of the most common techniques of anma and one of the primary techniques used in Japanese facial massage, especially when using lubrication. The light stroking is used to improve circulation and relax the muscles.

In anma, *kei satsu ho* is most often performed without lubrication, but in Japanese facial massage it is often applied with lubrication. Regardless, it is important to apply very smooth strokes to increase the circulation and bring heat to the surface and to maintain the heat during the movement.

Light-stroking technique can be applied with various parts of the hand that are usually chosen for the best fit to the parts of the body and the purpose of the technique. The techniques most often used in Japanese facial massage for stroking the face are:

1. stroking with the entire hand
   (*shu sho kei satsu ho*)
2. stroking with the flat part of the thumb
   (*so shi kei satsu ho*)
3. stroking with the tip of the thumb
   (*bo shi to kei satsu ho*)
4. stroking with the base of the thumb (thenar)
   (*bo shi kyu kei satsu ho*)
5. stroking with the side of the hand (hypothenar)
   (*ko shi kyu kei satsu ho*)
6. stroking with the flat parts of four fingers
   (*shi shi kei satsu ho*)
7. stroking with the flat part of two fingers
   (*ni shi kei satsu ho*)
8. stroking with the tips of two fingers
   (*ni shi to kei satsu ho*)

Here are some important tips and precautionary notes you should know. Your wrists, elbows, and shoulders must be relaxed and loose enough to adjust easily to the contours of the face and neck. Tense shoulders and elbows make for a jerky and uncomfortable application. You can increase the pressure of the stroking after the tissue is properly warmed, but do not use extreme pressure with this technique. Stroking must be applied smoothly and rhythmically. Your fingers must be kept together to ensure that the heat is kept on the surface of the skin.

2. Kneading Technique—*Ju Netsu Ho*

Kneading technique, or *ju netsu ho*, is the primary technique used in anma, but it is less often used in Japanese facial massage. However, *ju netsu ho* is the primary technique when working on the neck without using a lubricant. This is because the application of *ju netsu ho* is limited when you are unable to grasp the surface, and when lubricant is used it becomes even more difficult to apply. If you are accustomed to applying the kneading techniques of Swedish massage, these techniques might seem similar, but they are actually very different.

揉捏法

Ju netsu ho

揉捻法

(Also known as *ju nen ho*)

The main purpose of *ju netsu ho* is to reduce the tension of the muscles. The two primary application types of *ju netsu ho* are kneading and rotating. Kneading is usually applied through the continuous motion of squeezing and releasing the muscle between your fingers and the thumb or palm, similar to kneading bread dough, and is often used with neck massage. Rotation is applied by anchoring a portion of the hand to the surface and applying circular motions without sliding over the skin. When you are kneading or rotating, pay close attention to the condition of the muscles to detect any kind of irregular tightness.

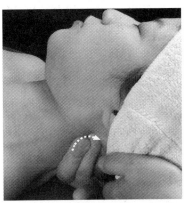
Kneading while squeezing

There are many ways to apply *ju netsu ho*, including techniques which do not contain kneading or rotating movements. For example, you can knead by pushing the muscle between two alternating thumbs, or by using very small, alternating strokes with the edges of the thumbs.

The following are the *ju netsu ho* applications most often used in Japanese facial massage:

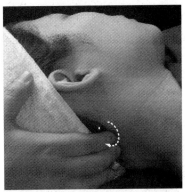
Two finger rotations

1. kneading with a squeezing movement
   (*ha aku ju netsu ho*)
2. kneading with the flat part of the thumb
   (*bo shi ju netsu ho*)
3. kneading with the tip of the thumb
   (*bo shi to ju netsu ho*)
4. kneading with the tips of two fingers
   (*ni shi to ju netsu ho*)
5. kneading with the tips of three fingers
   (*san shi to ju netsu ho*)

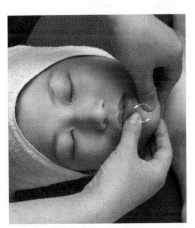
Kneading with the tips of the thumbs

3. Vibration Technique—*Shin Sen Ho*

振せん法

Shin sen ho

Vibration technique, or *shin sen ho*, may sound simple, but developing fine control in your palms and fingers takes time and practice. This can be the most difficult technique to master. Proficiency may take years, but your ability will improve with practice.

Unlike stroking or kneading techniques that work on the surface, vibration aims to work deeper into the muscle. Practitioners often alternate between vibration and kneading. The combination has two benefits: they loosen muscles more effectively, and the hands will not tire as quickly. *Shin sen ho* is also often combined with *ap paku ho* (pressure technique, see next page). If a client finds that *ap paku ho* is a little painful, vibration can be used to disperse the painful pressure over a larger area of muscle.

There are two different ways to apply vibration: inner and outer. The distinction between them lies not in the position of the hand but in the type of movement you use to vibrate. The two techniques have different purposes, and it is important to develop control of the depth, length, and speed of the vibrations. As with *ju netsu ho*, some practice is required to master this technique.

内振

I. Inner vibration

With inner vibration, the point is to send fine, concentrated vibrational force into the inner layers of the muscle. Inner vibration is usually applied by tensing the entire upper body and sending the vibration from deep within your body. There should be little vibrational movement at the point of contact.

外振

II. Outer vibration

Outer vibration is used to loosen muscles on the surface of an area. While applying outer vibration, your upper body should remain loose and relaxed. Outer vibration is usually applied by using vigorous vibrations at the place of contact and does not require the same level of concentration or vibrational force as inner vibration does.

Generally speaking, beginning students should not use the vibration technique on the face; it is uncomfortable for the client unless you have mastered this technique, but it is excellent for the neck and other parts of the body. When applying the vibration technique on the neck, it is usually applied using inner vibration, rather than outer vibration, due to the proximity to the head.

4. Pressure Technique—*Ap Paku Ho*

Pressure technique, or *ap paku ho*, can be applied in many different ways, using any amount of force or for any duration of time. Generally, only gentle, light pressure is used on the face. *Ap paku ho* is very similar to *o atsu ho*, the primary pressure technique in shiatsu. Anma practitioners who specialized and used this technique for full-body massage early in this century began calling themselves shiatsu therapists.

圧迫法

Ap paku ho

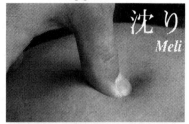

沈り
Meli

Strength of Pressure (*Meli* and *Kali*)

The amount of force you apply requires you to change the angle of your thumb in relation to the surface of the body. With heavy pressure, you must be closer to the fingertip to support a much more defined pressure, while a flat thumb is softer and does not require this support. *Meli* and *kali* are the Japanese terms used to describe the different types of pressure used in Japanese facial massage.

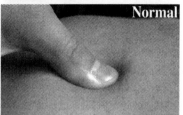

Normal

Meli literally means "sink" in Japanese. It uses the tip of the thumb (or fingers) to sink deeply into the skin. *Meli* is usually deep, heavy pressure for longer durations, used in conjunction with breathing and is often used for sedation (*sha* in Japanese) with fewer deep, long applications.

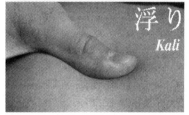

浮り
Kali

Kali literally means "floating" in Japanese. It uses light pressure with a flat finger or fingers held parallel to the skin surface. *Kali* is usually of shorter duration with more frequent applications. The breathing cycle is not as important. It is often used for tonifying (*ho* in Japanese).

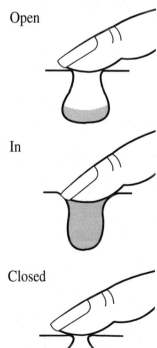

Open

In

Closed

Applying Pressure to the Acupoints (*Tsubo*)

This method is only used to stimulate the acupoints on the meridians (*kei ketsu* in Japanese) to tonify or sedate the meridians. You must pay attention to the client's breathing cycle when applying pressure to the *kei ketsu*. As you press a *tsubo*, imagine three steps. First, imagine opening the *tsubo* with light pressure to make the body aware that you are going to stimulate it. Then, imagine entering into that *tsubo* as you press. This step requires strong pressure over a longer duration of time to stimulate the *tsubo*. Finally, imagine closing the *tsubo* using slightly lighter pressure as the previous step and for the same duration. Closing is very important because it ensures that the *tsubo* is not left exposed.

5. Percussion Technique—*Ko Da Ho*

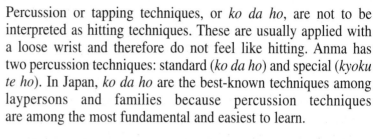

Ko da ho

Percussion or tapping techniques, or *ko da ho*, are not to be interpreted as hitting techniques. These are usually applied with a loose wrist and therefore do not feel like hitting. Anma has two percussion techniques: standard (*ko da ho*) and special (*kyoku te ho*). In Japan, *ko da ho* are the best-known techniques among laypersons and families because percussion techniques are among the most fundamental and easiest to learn.

Ko da ho is applied lightly and rapidly by tapping the face with different parts of your hand. The hand retains the same shape during the percussion, with your shoulder and elbow fairly loose and flexible. Percussion is usually applied by alternating both hands, but it can be applied with just one hand for application on the face.

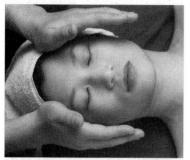

Ko da ho penetrates the facial layers more deeply than other Japanese facial-massage techniques. Other techniques such as kneading or stroking tend to affect only the surface of the face, but percussion can stimulate the deepest layers of the tissue. It also gently stimulates the facial nerves so that circulation of the blood can be increased.

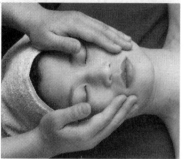

Percussion with flat fingers

Because of the size and shape of the face, only a few types of percussion are effective. *Ko da ho* can be used on the face and the neck but must be applied very gently, especially when working with the face. These are the techniques that work well on the face:

1. flat part of four fingers   (*shi shi ko da ho*)
2. tips of four fingers   (*shi shi to ko da ho*)
3. tips of the fingers   (*shi to ko da ho*)
4. flat part of thumb   (*bo shi ko da ho*)

The following two techniques are often used on the neck only:

5. back of the four fingers   (*shu hai ko da ho*)
6. side of the closed hand   (*shu kan ko da ho*)

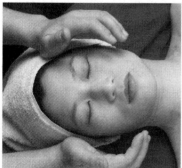

Begin by practicing these techniques slowly until they are smooth and rhythmic. Try to get into a triplet rhythm, where you are skipping the second beat. The key is to control your hands whether you are using hard or soft bounces. It is important to develop your sensitivity to adjust to your client's requirements. This technique should not be applied too forcefully, using just enough force to be effective. With time, you will develop a sense of how much force to apply.

Percussion with tips of fingers

6. Special Percussion Technique—*Kyoku Te Ho*

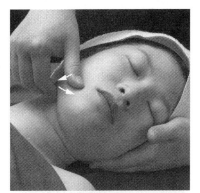

曲手法

Kyoku te ho

Special percussion technique, or *kyoku te ho*, is similar to *ko da ho* but is a unique way to perform percussion that is found only in anma. The difference between the two is that *ko da ho* is a simple percussion in which the hand does not change shape during the application. *Kyoku te ho* is a series of specially modified percussion techniques where the hand changes shape during each percussive movement. Also, *kyoku te ho* is typically a more gentle technique than *ko da ho*. *Kyoku te ho* requires a fair amount of practice for smooth integration with the other techniques.

Mawashi te of the *kyoku te ho* is the primary distinguishing technique that is an essential feature of Japanese facial massage.

Each technique in *kyoku te ho* is unique in application and effect. *Kyoku te ho* techniques are precise techniques designed to work very specific body regions; generally, a technique designed for one area does not work well on other parts of the body.

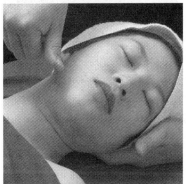

Thumb and finger flipping percussion

Improper application of *kyoku te ho* can create severe stress to the joints on the practitioner's fingers and wrists. Proper training is highly recommended for a better understanding of *kyoku te ho*. For more information about the application of *kyoku te ho* techniques, please refer to *Anma: The Art of Japanese Massage*. The following five techniques of *kyoku te ho* are presented in this book.

Two of the easiest and most common variations that can be applied to the face are:

1. thumb and finger flipping   (*mawashi te*)
2. two-handed paddle wheel inward   (*sukui te*)

For the head and scalp, two of the most common techniques are:

3. finger short stroking and jumping   (*tsumami te*)
4. slow pulling   (*yanagi te*)

A common technique for the neck:

5. two-handed paddle wheel stroking   (*sukui te*)

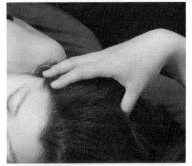

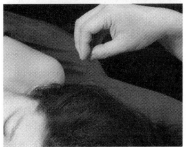

Stroking and jumping percussion

7. Stretch and Movement Technique—*Un Do Ho*

運動法

Un do ho

Stretch and movement techniques, or *un do ho*, are a series of techniques which involve movement, stretching, and exercise. These are considered slightly advanced techniques, and while none of *un do ho* techniques are immediately recognizable as massage-like, they are still categorized as a part of massage techniques. Although primarily used to work on the neck rather than the face, *un do ho* is an important part of anma and Japanese facial massage because, when used in combination with the other techniques, it greatly enhances the therapeutic value of the treatment.

These techniques are commonly used in Japan for rehabilitation of injuries, and *un do ho* is one of the oldest known techniques for rehabilitation. Modern Japanese rehabilitation techniques came from this tradition.

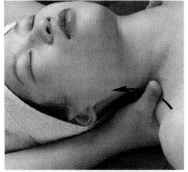

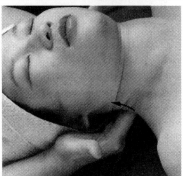

The purpose of movement and stretching is slightly different than the goals of other facial-massage techniques. Each individual technique in *un do ho* has a different purpose. Stretching the muscles, aligning the structure, and regaining or maintaining the range of motion of the joint are the chief goals.

The majority of *un do ho* techniques can generally be categorized into five different groups of techniques. These are:

1. movement by the client alone
    (*ji do un do ho*)
2. adjustment techniques
    (*kyo sei ho*)
3. movement by the therapist
    (*ta do un do ho*)
4. stretching techniques
    (*shin cho un do ho*)
5. exercising movement through resistance
    (*tei ko un do ho*)

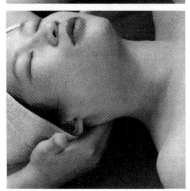

Stretching the neck

Un do ho must be applied very carefully and gently. Most of the techniques require you to work slowly as well. It is also very important to incorporate your client's breathing cycle into the application. Some techniques are advanced and require classroom instruction and a solid understanding of anatomy and physiology.

The previous seven techniques are the traditional anma techniques. Traditionally, anma is known as containing seven application techniques, but in reality, there are many techniques in anma that do not belong to these categories. A few of these are listed below as supplemental techniques.

8. *Kyo Satsu Ho*

強擦法
Kyo satsu ho

This is a stroking and rotating technique like *kei satsu ho,* but it uses much heavier pressure. It is also called *an netsu ho.* There are two ways which *kyo satsu ho* can be applied. Small rotations can be applied to the joint with heavy pressure, or you can stroke with heavy pressure using the thumb. *Kyo satsu ho* is not a commonly-used technique and is usually applied to reduce pain and stiffness, as well as to improve mobility of the joints. This technique is especially useful for conditions affecting the temporomandibular joint (TMJ).

9. *Ha Aku Ho*

把握法
Ha aku ho

This squeezing or grabbing technique is generally combined with other techniques such as stroking, vibration, or rotating to aid in the application. For example, *ha aku ho* and *kei satsu ho* can be combined to become *ha aku kei satsu ho* (stroking while squeezing). *Ha aku ho* is not often used alone to work on the face. The difference between *ha aku ho* and *ap paku ho* is that *ha aku ho* squeezes from two directions simultaneously and *ap paku ho* applies pressure from only one direction. Although rarely used for facial massage, this technique is very effective and used occasionally in Japanese facial massage directly over the TMJ to reduce tension in the jaw. This technique is commonly used in neck massage.

10. *Ken Biki Ho*

This pulling and applying tension technique is rarely used by itself on the face but is often used when working on the neck. It is generally used to lightly stretch by pulling or to apply tension to the muscle in combination with another technique for enhanced effects.

11. *Shin Ken Ho*

This special stretching technique is an advanced technique that is used in Japanese facial massage only on the inside of the mouth and also on the neck. It is useful in situations where you must manually force the muscles or fascia to stretch or to free unwanted adhesion in the tissues. It is usually applied to regions with limited mobility that are difficult to stretch.

12. Shiatsu Techniques

Shiatsu began to develop as a separate massage method in the early 1900s as an outgrowth from anma, which included shiatsu techniques but was categorized simply as a form of anma. Shiatsu continued to evolve as an independent method of massage study, and in 1964 it became formally recognized as a separate massage modality. Since shiatsu originally was a part of anma, most shiatsu techniques are very similar to anma, and large portions of the applications overlap each other. Most of the techniques used in Japanese facial massage come from anma, but a few are taken from the current techniques that are basic to the practice of shiatsu.

The techniques have similarities between them, yet the method of application is quite different. The primary difference between anma and shiatsu is that anma is a kneading-based therapy, and shiatsu is a pressure-based therapy. While anma combines a diverse range of techniques, shiatsu relies primarily on the use of pressure application and seldom includes other techniques.

The following five techniques are used in shiatsu practice:

1. *o atsu ho*
This push and pressure technique is the pressure technique of shiatsu. It is the same technique as *ap paku ho* of anma but relies more on the thumb. Many pressure techniques in the energizing stage (Chapter 9) can also be considered as shiatsu techniques.

2. *an netsu ho*
This technique is identical to *kyo satsu ho* of anma, but shiatsu practitioners call it *an netsu ho*.

3. *shin do ho*
This is a vibration technique used in shiatsu. In anma, it is called *shin sen ho*. They are the same technique, although more pressure is usually applied with *shin do ho*.

4. *bu satsu ho*
This is technically the same as *kei satsu ho* from anma, although it is usually applied with slightly more pressure. It is commonly used on the abdomen.

5. *shin ten ho*
This is a stretching technique used in shiatsu. It is identical to *ta do un do ho* and *shin cho un do ho* of the *un do ho* techniques in anma.

Meanings of the Symbols Used in this Book

To accompany the written explanations, I have placed several types of arrows over the pictures to help explain different types of movement visually. The different types of arrows show different types of movement or pressure made while applying Japanese facial massage. Familiarity with the symbols listed below aids you in understanding this book.

Bold straight arrows
These arrows show the direction of stroking to slide over the surface of the skin. This arrow mainly indicates *kei satsu ho* or *kyo satsu ho*.

Dotted straight arrows
These arrows show the direction of pressure or movement that grips skin and muscle, which way to pull or push, or just the direction of applied pressure for techniques such as *ju netsu ho*, *ap paku ho*, and *ha aku ho*. The dotted arrow means that your hands should remain in the same position relative to the skin and not move over the skin.

Bold circular arrows
These arrows show the direction of circular stroking, mainly in *kei satsu ho*. This movement slides over the skin or the clothes.

Dotted circular arrows
These arrows show the direction of rotation or circular movement that grips the muscle or skin, without moving over the skin. Your hand moves just slightly in the direction of the applied pressure such as with *ju netsu ho* and *kyo satsu ho*. The three-quarter circle and some of the half-circles show continuing rotation. The one-quarter circle and the rest of the half-circle arrows show movement. Refer to the instructions in the text for each case.

Zig-zag arrows
These arrows show vibration. The direction of the arrow shows the direction of the pressure you apply with the vibration.

Three-dimensional arrows
These arrows show movement of the body. This arrow is also used to indicate a direction of pressure that could be difficult to demonstrate with a two-dimensional arrow.

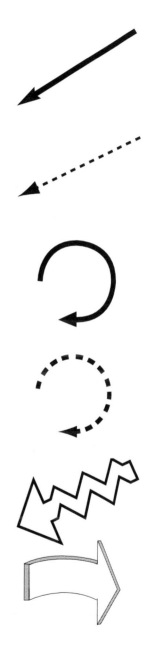

Chapter Seven
MASSAGE TECHNIQUES FOR THE NECK

In this chapter, I introduce five basic examples of massage techniques for the neck. The focus of the chapter is on how to give a smooth and relaxing, yet therapeutic, neck massage before applying a facial massage. These are five examples of neck-massage techniques most commonly used in conjunction with Japanese facial massage. These techniques require the use of lubricant and are used for improving the fluid circulation to the face, as well as for relaxing the client. These techniques should be applied before a facial massage. Neck-massage techniques can be used in daily life with family and friends—they are beneficial skills for anyone to learn.

If you are applying a facial massage as a part of a full-body routine, the facial massage is more calm and relaxed than the back and shoulder work. The goal here is to relax the client, release tension in the neck, and increase the blood circulation to the face, rather than using a deep therapeutic approach to correct a neck problem.

The client should be on his or her back, and the practitioner should be seated directly behind the client's head. You can also add anma techniques to enhance the neck massage. Carefully adjust the amount of pressure that you apply to accommodate the sensitivity of your client. You will find that many people have a great deal of tension in the neck. Neck work must always be done with caution, using moderate pressure. I would suggest not working on the neck for more than fifteen minutes at a time. If a person needs attention on the neck for more than fifteen minutes, have the client come back another day. If possible, it is best to work on the shoulders and upper back before working on the neck, since neck stress often originates in those areas.

Close Relation Between the Neck and Face

Stress is the main cause of various illnesses. Many people carry stress in the neck and shoulder regions. This can lead to various types of discomfort and health problems such as headaches, frozen shoulders, facial neuralgia, and facial paralysis. The proper application of a neck massage can make a noticeable difference in the physical and psychological reduction of stress.

Tight neck muscles restrict blood flow to the face and can limit mobility of the head. Tight facial muscles can be caused by tight neck muscles because they work so closely together. Often tight facial muscles will not loosen until the neck tightness is released. Tight muscles in both neck and face can restrict the proper blood flow essential for facial skin to stay healthy. Blood carries oxygen, nutrition, and minerals, while removing toxins and unwanted oils throughout the body. Proper circulation of the blood is essential to replenish the body and prevent premature aging of the skin.

A ten-minute neck massage can be as beneficial as an entire facial massage. Neck massage is an important compliment to facial massage, and it is an important part of the facial treatment. A tight neck can limit the results of even the best facial-massage application. Also, neck massage can prevent the possibility of the client getting a headache when you reach the energizing stage of the facial massage. Neck massage encourages proper lymph flow in the neck, increasing the opportunity for toxins to drain from the face. Otherwise, toxins may stay in the face and settle in the neck region.

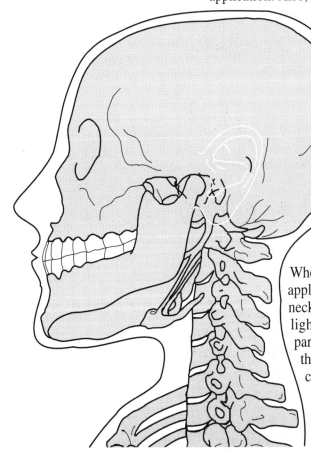

The neck has a relatively complex muscle and bone construction. The illustration to the left is a side skeletal view to show the bone construction of the neck. All neck massage must be applied properly and cautiously.

When working on the neck, the practitioner can apply fairly strong pressure on the back of the neck, medium pressure on the sides, and relatively light pressure on the front of the neck. In particular, when massaging the front of the neck, the practitioner must be especially sensitive and careful with the amount of pressure applied.

Application of Neck Massage

All neck (and facial) massages can be applied with the client wearing a loose-fitting shirt, preferably with a wide neck. It is easiest to apply massage with a sheet or towel draped to cover the chest area without a shirt being worn. Be sure the client is properly covered to keep the body warm.

Practice the neck massage until you can comfortably and confidently apply each technique. If you feel nervous, especially when working very close to the client's head, the client is likely to notice and feel uncomfortable with your nervousness. Techniques with lighter pressure should always begin the routine, followed by techniques that require heavier pressure.

All techniques should be applied to a degree relatively comfortable to the client. The client should only feel a slight discomfort if he or she has a very tight neck or pain in the neck area. To help the client stay relaxed, the practitioner should also be relaxed and move around as little as possible. None of these techniques require the practitioner to stand up or move from side to side. When the practitioner is trying to relax the client, all the strokes must be performed at a slow rate. When applying really deep strokes, you must slow down your movements.

Head Positions for Facial and Neck Massage

When massaging the face and neck, there are two preferred positions to use for the placement of the head.

Center position
In this position, the nose should be pointed upward toward the ceiling, even with the median line of the body. This position is used for working on the areas in the middle of the face such as the chin and nose. Most of the neck massage is done in this head position.

Center Position

45° tilt position
In this position, the nose should make a 45° angle out from the center median line of the body. This position is used to massage from the side of the nose to just below the eyes, the cheeks, the middle of the jawbone, the ears, and the temples.

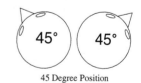

45 Degree Position

It is good to rotate the head a little during some techniques. As everyone's facial contours are different, you'll need to adjust the rotation accordingly to give yourself proper access to a particular region. This is best done by cupping the base of the skull and gently turning it to the side as needed. It is best to group techniques together on one side of the head at a time to minimize the frequency of rotation.

Japanese Facial-Massage Techniques—Example #1

Up-Stroking on the Side of the Neck

Japanese name for this technique

四指軽擦法

(ryo) shi shi kei satsu ho

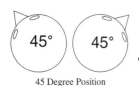

45 Degree Position

The purpose of this technique

Reduce neck tension and improve circulation and *ki* flow in the neck and base of the skull

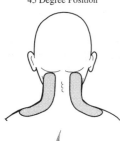

Area of application

On the sides of the neck (scalenes and sternocleidomastoid) and at the base of the skull

Generous Lubrication

Description

The next five techniques for massaging the neck are applied with lubrication. More lubrication is useful for large, fast movements and less is advisable for smaller, slower movements. Oil can be used, but is often messy even in the hands of an expert, so lotion is recommended.

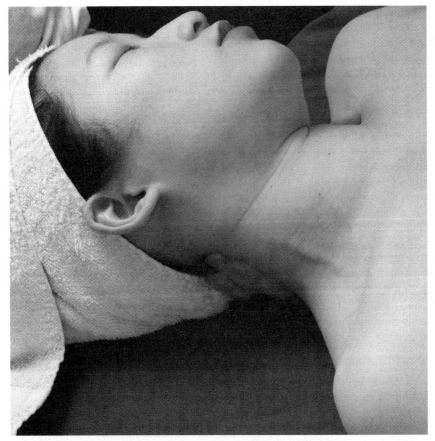

1 Grasp the client's neck at the base of the skull with your left hand. The thumb should remain on the other side of the neck. Turn the head slightly for easier access to the neck.

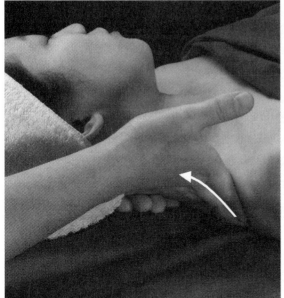

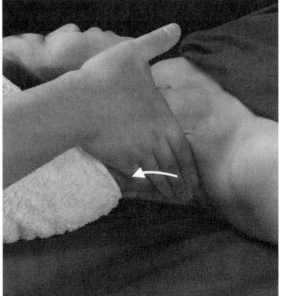

2 Slide the fingers under the shoulder blade (over the AC joint). Using the side of the index finger, push the shoulder toward the ceiling by turning your wrist. Turn the wrist farther to stroke the back of the shoulder with the index and middle fingers, moving toward the crook of the neck.

3 As you reach the bottom of the neck, turn the wrist more parallel to the neck and use the flat parts of the fingers to stroke the back of the neck toward the base of the skull. Meanwhile, slide your left hand under the spine as far as it can reach, placing the tip of the index finger between the spine and right scapular.

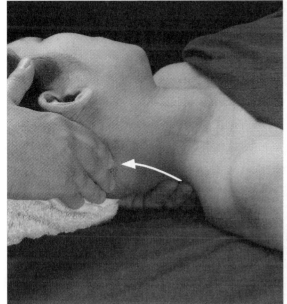

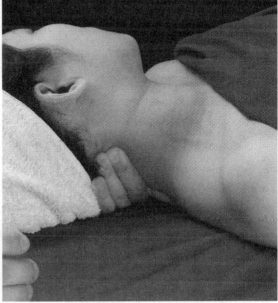

4 As your right hand reaches the base of the skull, stroke the side of the neck with the flat parts of the fingers of the left hand, from between the vertebrae and the scapula toward the base of the skull.

5 While the left hand is stroking, remove the right hand from the head. As your left hand finishes stroking, place the right hand under the scapula and repeat entire procedure for fifteen to thirty seconds. Repeat on other side of the neck.

Japanese Facial-Massage Techniques—Example #2

Light Stroking up the Front of the Neck

Japanese name for this technique

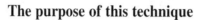

shu sho kei satsu ho

0°

Center Position

The purpose of this technique

Increase the blood flow to the face

Area of application

Front of the neck, from the clavicle region to the chin

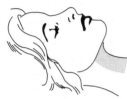

Description

Start massaging the front of the neck with this gentle up-stroking technique. It is an excellent technique for increasing blood circulation to the face, as well as for relaxing the neck and releasing tension. You can either apply with both hands at the same time or by alternating hands as demonstrated here. It is important to keep your hands and wrists loose to easily follow the contours of the neck. Relax your arms and shoulders as well.

Generous Lubrication

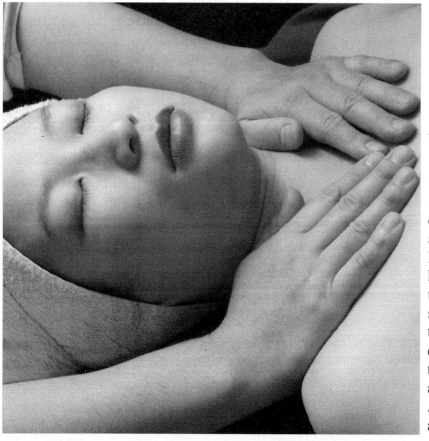

1 The client's head should be in the center position. Using a generous amount of lubrication on your hands, gently place the hands on both sides of the neck with the fingers over the collar bone, pointed toward each other at about a 90° angle. Again, keep your arms and shoulders relaxed.

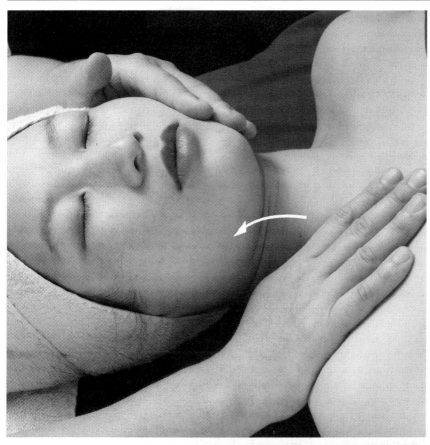

2 Start gently stroking with the right hand from the collar bone toward the neck. Your hand should be relaxed. Fit the palm and side of the fingers to the contour of the neck by slowly turning them toward you as you stroke. Do not apply any pressure to the neck, as the weight of the hand is more than sufficient for this pressure. Finish the stroke as you reach the jaw.

3 As you finish stroking with the right hand, start stroking with the left hand in the same fashion. As your left hand finishes the stroke, start again with the right hand and continue alternating hands as you stroke. Maintain plenty of lubrication so you do not pull the skin during the application, and keep your strokes fairly slow. Repeat for fifteen to thirty seconds or for as long as you desire.

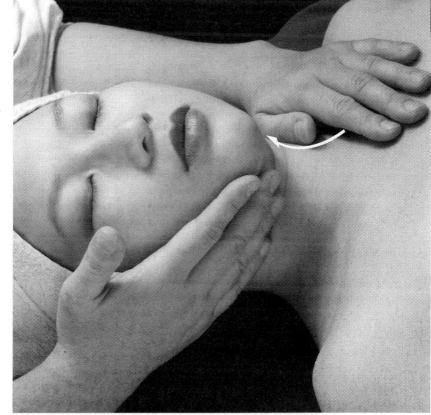

Stroking under the Chin

Japanese name for this technique

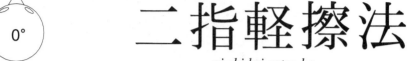

二指軽擦法

ni shi kei satsu ho

Center Position

The purpose of this technique

Help improve the appearance under the chin

Area of application

Under the chin (mandible)

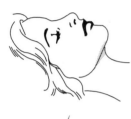

Description

This and the following technique (Example #4) are commonly combined, alternating one after another, for an effective way to massage under the chin. The application should be very smooth, with your shoulders and elbows relaxed. As you become more familiar with this technique, you can include a movement of the upper shoulder to create a much smoother application than with the fingers alone.

Generous Lubrication

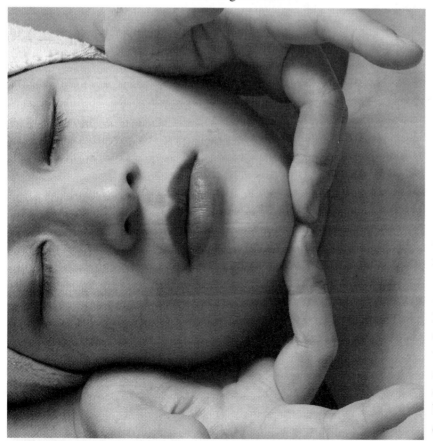

1 Gently rest the heels of your hands in front of the client's ears so the fingers are relaxed and have easy access to the chin. Put as little pressure on the face as possible, using only enough pressure to keep the hands steady. Place the middle and ring fingers of both hands under the chin at the center.

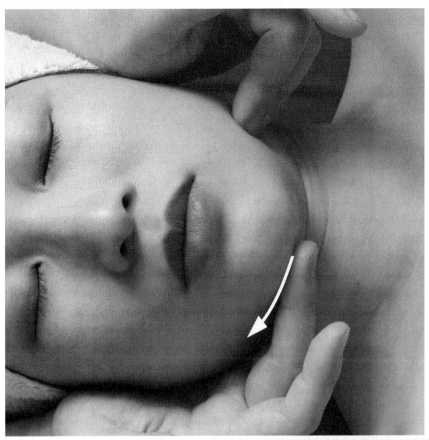

2 Begin gently stroking under the chin with the middle and ring fingers of the right hand, following the line of the jaw. The heel of the hand can remain in front of the ear while you stroke, or you can drop it down over the ear for a smoother stroking movement. Stop stroking once you reach the back of the ear.

3 As you finish stroking with the right hand, begin stroking with the left hand in the same fashion. As your left hand finishes the stroke, start again with the right hand and continue to use alternating hands as you stroke. Maintain plenty of lubrication so you do not pull the skin. Keep your strokes slow and smooth. Repeat for ten to fifteen seconds or for as long as desired.

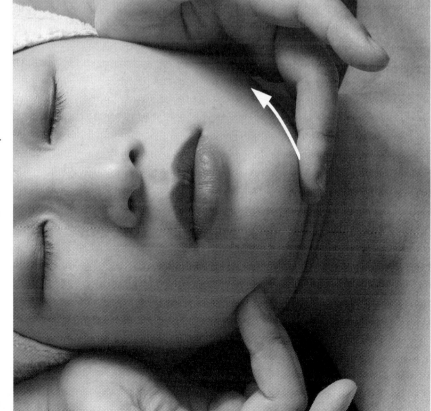

Japanese Facial-Massage Techniques—Example #4

Paddle Percussion under the Chin

Japanese name for this technique

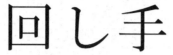

mawashi te (kyoku te ho)

The purpose of this technique

Improve the appearance under the chin

Area of application

Under the chin (mandible)

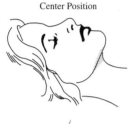

Center Position

Description

This example uses a very light and soothing percussion technique under the chin and is often combined with the previous technique to create a very effective way to work under the chin. The percussion is very light, yet generally uses faster movement. This technique does not pound into the underside of the chin, but rather uses sweeping strokes to create percussion with the tip of the fingers.

Generous Lubrication

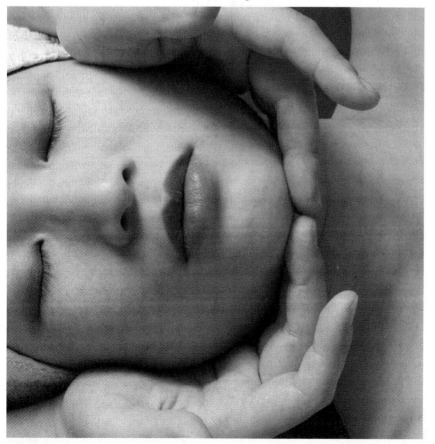

1 Use the same starting hand positions as in the previous example.

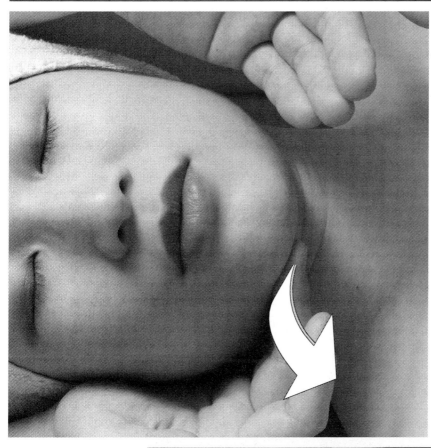

2 Begin sliding under the chin with the flat part of the index and ring fingers. Stroke up toward the ceiling in a sweeping fashion while rotating the entire hand and wrist. Pressure into the chin must be kept to a minimum.

3 As you finish sweeping the right hand, begin sweep-stroking with the left hand in the same fashion. As your left hand finishes the stroke, start again with the right hand, and continue using alternating hands to create a paddle-wheel stroke. You no longer need to rest the hand on the face at this point; both hands can stay in the air. Move the application to both the left and right to cover the entire bottom of the chin.

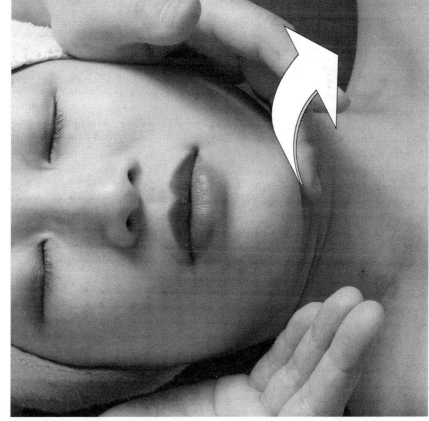

Japanese Facial-Massage Techniques—Example #5

Light Stroking up the Side of the Neck

Japanese name for this technique

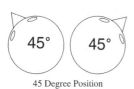

45 Degree Position

手掌軽擦法

shu sho kei satsu ho

The purpose of this technique

Increase blood circulation to the face

Area of application

From the side of the neck to the cheek

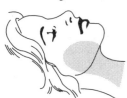

Description

Generous Lubrication

This technique is similar to Example #2 but uses a more rapid up-stroking on one side of the face at a time, with the head turned about 45° to the side for easier access to the neck. This example is generally used to start a facial massage in combination with the facial techniques that are demonstrated in the next chapter. It is best to apply this technique during both cleansing and moisturizing stages.

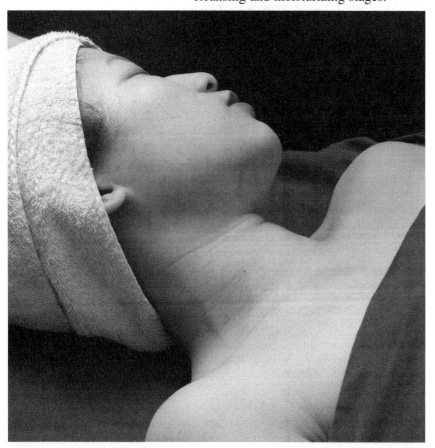

1 Gently turn the head about 45° to the left.

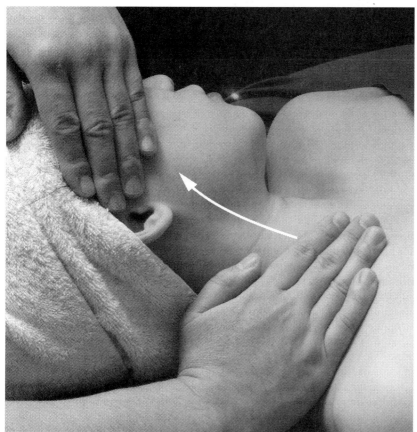

2 Place your left hand in front of the ear to stabilize the head. Place the right hand at the bottom of the neck over the collar bone, bringing the hand in at a shallow angle so it does not slap into the skin. Start stroking the front and side of the neck (over the sternocleidomastoid muscle) and continue up to the side of the cheek. Stop once you reach the cheek bone (zygomatic arch). Your hand should be relaxed, with the palm and sides of the fingers fitting to the contour of the client's neck.

3 As the right hand finishes the stroke, place the left hand at the same starting position and stroke over the same path. The left hand can move slightly into the medial side of the cheek. Alternate your hands to create continuous stroking for improving circulation to the face. Continue for about fifteen to thirty seconds, then repeat on the other side of the neck.

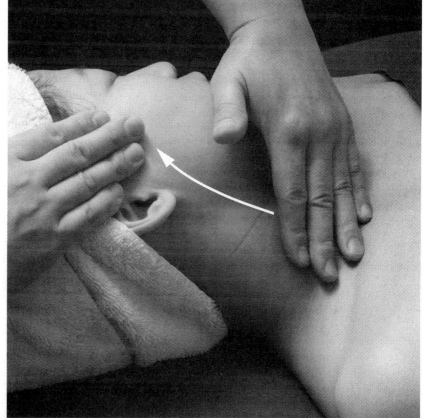

Chapter Eight

BASIC JAPANESE FACIAL-MASSAGE TECHNIQUES

In this chapter, I introduce twenty examples of the most commonly used techniques in Japanese facial massage. The techniques given in this chapter were selected because they are easy to learn and apply. There are many techniques used in traditional Japanese facial massage, but these twenty represent the core techniques that every student must master before moving to more advanced techniques. Using these techniques you can give an excellent full facial massage. Advanced techniques very often address specific conditions, such as sinus blockage or inflammation of the Temporomandibular Joint (TMJ) and are not frequently used otherwise. At least ninety percent of every advanced facial massage session consists of these fundamental techniques, so it is necessary to learn them first and master them thoroughly.

Massage is not about how many different techniques you know, but how well and how smoothly you can apply the simple fundamental techniques. The most important skills in massage therapy, especially at the professional level, are smoothness of technical application and seamless joining of one technique to the next. Each technique must be properly mastered at the outset, and from there one goes on to the development of sequence, blending one technique into the next without breaking the rhythm. For the massage to have a therapeutic effect, your body must be relaxed and confident in the application of the strokes—this is essential, and it only comes after thorough assimilation of the techniques. Learn these foundational strokes completely and achieve this relaxation. The client will have a very hard time relaxing to the massage if the practitioner is not relaxed in this way.

Japanese Facial-Massage Procedure

In Chapters 7 through 10, I introduce forty-five examples of neck and face techniques in the order in which they are often performed. It is important to arrange these techniques according to the needs of the client. A variety of techniques can work together for a full massage.

I do not believe in teaching a regimented massage routine that must be followed step by step. As massage is used at the therapeutic level, you must carefully understand the condition of your client and utilize the techniques best suited for their individual needs. There is no routine that works best for everyone. As every body has different conditions which must be considered, every face also introduces a variety of conditions requiring special attention. Such conditions are: how oily or dry the skin is, the different contours of the facial structure, sensitivities of the skin, age and ethnic background (where you find different densities of the muscles). To address these factors, you must modify your technique and routine and utilize the best techniques for each individual. It takes time to develop this sense and determine what is proper for each condition in massage.

Another reason I do not teach an exact routine is because students get in the habit of using only that routine. Massage therapy is not an assembly-line job: massage therapists must be creative and thoughtful. Know the conditions of each client's face and adjust the massage to create an individualized routine. Massage is an art, like creating a painting, and I like to show the different techniques as I would introduce different colors on a palette. But, if I tell you how or what to paint, it becomes no longer your art. Also, I encourage massage therapists to combine knowledge of other existing massage techniques with those in this book to create their own art. Feel free to modify any of the techniques in this book, so long as they do not negatively effect the client.

There are many ways to arrange the techniques for a Japanese facial massage. In order to give you a preliminary understanding, I introduce a general routine that follows the most traditional sequence of the techniques. Again, the massage you give depends on each client, but I offer some general guidelines for students to practice with. A smooth, polished facial massage will come with practice; as you develop your own style of massage, your facial massage skills will mature into an organic part of your own repertoire.

Japanese facial massage often begins with a gentle neck massage (introduced in a previous chapter). This helps to release muscle tension in the back of the neck and improve blood flow to the face, which are essential for improving facial appearance and preventing wrinkles and age spots. Neck massage, as used in Japanese facial massage, averages three to five minutes unless the client requires more work.

After massaging the back of the neck, steam the face with warm moist towels for one or two minutes. If your hands are oily from the neck massage, wash your hands during this time, as oily hands disturb the cleanser, preventing it from foaming. Wrap the hair with a towel so the excess cleanser or moisturizer does not get into the hair. If there is any facial makeup, gently remove it with an astringent.

Next, for the cleansing stage, tilt the head to about 45°and begin massage on the front of the neck, lubricating with cleanser. Massage one side of the face, and then tilt the head to the other side and massage the face on that side with the same procedure. When this is completed, move the head to center position and massage the central part of the face. These techniques can be applied one after another to cover the entire face, but you can arrange them in whatever sequence you desire. Combine the strokes as befits the client, but do so smoothly so that the massage feels like an integrated treatment, rather than a series of techniques strung together.

To begin the moisturizing stage, carefully remove the cleanser from the client's face with a moist towel. At this point you can steam the face again if you wish. Repeat the entire massage procedure as used in the cleansing stage, this time using moisturizer as lubricant. The cleansing stage is the largest part of the Japanese facial massage; the moisturizing stage, although the same routine, takes only half as long. When the moisturizer begins to feel sticky under your fingers, it is time to complete the moisturizing stage.

After the moisturizing stage, the facial massage continues with the energizing stage. This procedure is covered in Chapter 9. Apply the strokes to stimulate the meridians and *tsubo* (acupoints). This balances the *ki* (energy) flow of the face and gives a natural face-lift effect.

After the energizing stage, apply the series of light lymph-draining strokes to remove toxins from the face which have been brought to the surface by the massage. This gives a nice, calm finishing touch to the face. This procedure is covered in Chapter 10.

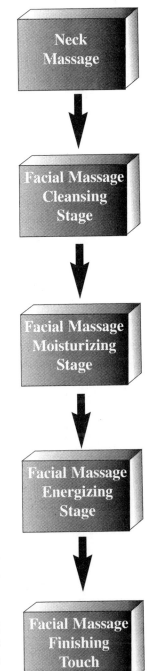

Before You Start

Before you begin Japanese facial massage, it is important to understand all application guidelines and precautions and also basic hand application techniques (see Chapters 5 and 6). If possible, wash your hands immediately before beginning the facial massage.

The client should lay on his or her back with the top of the head about six inches from the table's edge. If the client has long hair, it can fall over the edge of the table so that it is easier to do the neck massage. Cover the hair with a towel as explained on the following page. The client's hands can be placed at the sides or over the abdomen, whichever is more comfortable. Place a bolster or pillow under the knees for comfort, and drape the body with a sheet to maintain a suitable body temperature, adding a blanket if necessary. The client can wear a light shirt during the massage, but it is easier if their shoulders and neck are free of clothing.

The therapist should be seated (rather than kneeling) directly behind the head. The therapist should be able to apply all of these facial and neck massage techniques without having to stand up or move from side to side. To maximize relaxation of the client, the therapist needs to avoid all unnecessary movement, and for this purpose it is important to have everything necessary for Japanese facial massage prepared beforehand and put within reach (towels, cleanser, moisturizer, warm water, cottonballs, etc.). In the event the client has a skin reaction to the lubricant, it is good to have an extra set of moist towels nearby, so you may quickly remove it; extra towels are also handy for cleaning your own hands between stages.

A few Japanese facial-massage techniques do not require lubrication, but the majority of them do need at least some. In Japanese facial massage, it is always safer to overlubricate rather than to underlubricate and pull the skin.

Facial tissue is far more delicate than most other body regions and can be fatigued quickly. Practice these techniques with extra caution when learning, you must not overwork these tissues. Do not work the facial tissues longer than thirty minutes in a day, and no more than two or three times in a week. If you need more practice, find more people to practice on.

Bring the moisturizer and cleanser to room temperature before using them for facial massage.

How to Wrap the Towel

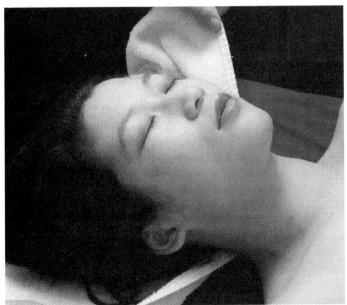

1 Slide one hand under the client's neck and bring the hand toward you until it is supporting the head. Lift the head gently and with your other hand slide the towel underneath, so the base of the skull is at the center of the towel's edge. Center the towel so there is an equal amount of towel on either side of the head.

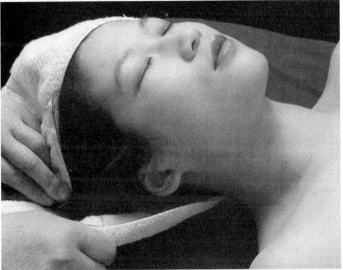

2 Bring the left side of the towel up and wrap it around (over) the head, with the edge of the towel covering the left ear and following the hairline at the top of the forehead as it continues down toward the table. Tuck a section of the towel in between the hair and the towel at the base of the head.

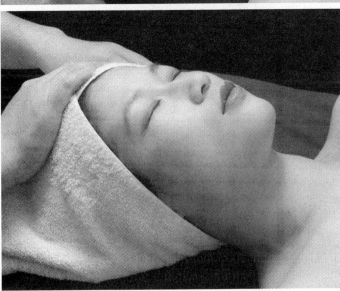

3 With your left hand, keep the towel tucked in, and use your right hand to wrap the right edge of the towel over the right ear and up along the hairline. You can use hair clips to hold the edges of the towel, or if the towel is big enough, you can wrap it around and tuck the edges under the head. Avoid using towels that are either too big or too small.

Japanese Facial-Massage Techniques—Example #6

Stroking up the Side of the Face

Japanese name for this technique

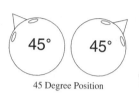

45 Degree Position

四指軽擦法

shi shi kei satsu ho

The purposes of this technique

Distribute lubrication over the cheek and increase circulation

Area of application

Over the entire cheek between the cheekbone and the jaw

Description

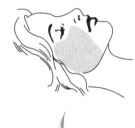

Generous Lubrication

Begin Japanese facial massage by applying a smooth, gentle, upward stroke on the cheek. This technique distributes the cleanser or moisturizer to the sides of the face and warms the tissues of the cheeks. It requires very subtle, even stroking with consistent pressure throughout the fingers. If you are applying this technique to a man with a beard, this stroke may go against the grain of his whiskers and cause slight discomfort; therefore, if the beard is very thick, you may skip over it and work just the upper cheeks. If you choose to work over the beard, stroke very slowly and adjust the application as needed. Do not apply moisturizer over facial hair.

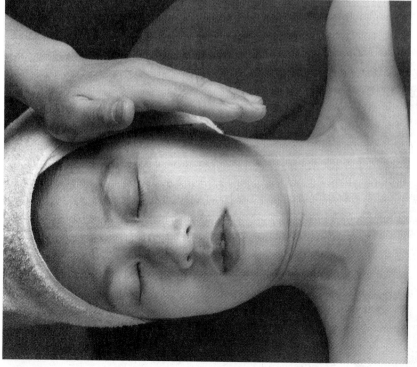

1 This technique begins with the head tilted to one side at about 45°, but you can choose to work with the head in the center position. Either way, work one cheek at a time. Gently place the heel of your left hand on the temple just above the left ear. Lightly cup the hand over the ear to support the head during the application of this technique.

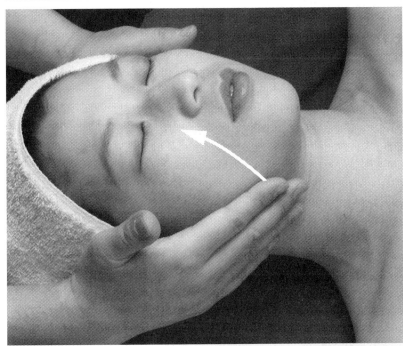

2 Gently place fingers on the edge of the jaw, in line with the natural crease between the nose and outer edge of mouth (nasolabial groove). Begin stroking lightly upward across the cheek from the jaw, using the flattened underside of the fingers. The fingertips follow the line of the nasolabial groove. This stroke is initially directed toward the side of the nose but gradually contours upward toward the cheekbone.

3 This stroke uses the entire hand as a unit, with the motion coming from the wrist and elbow—the fingers do not move on their own. Use the flattened underside of the fingers to provide even pressure against the entire cheek. Stroke until your fingertips reach the edge of the cheekbone, keeping your palm close to the face. Repeat several times, maintaining enough lubricant so the stroke does not pull the facial skin.

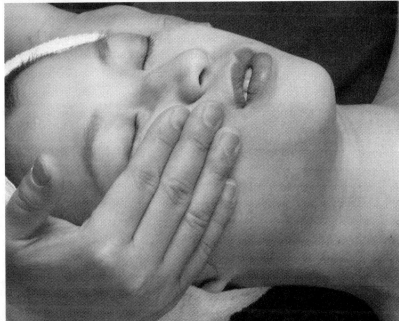

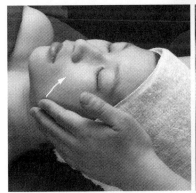
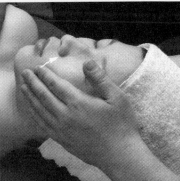
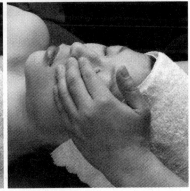

Japanese Facial-Massage Techniques—Example #7

Stroking up the Side of the Face with Both Hands

Japanese name for this technique

四指軽擦法

(ryo) shi shi kei satsu ho

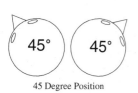

45 Degree Position

The purpose of this technique

Increase circulation and warm facial tissues

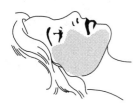

Area of application

Over the entire cheek between cheekbone and jaw

Generous Lubrication

Description

This is very similar to the previous example except that instead of a single hand providing the stroke, both hands are used for coordinated alternating strokes. Again, use plenty of lubrication to avoid pulling the facial skin (it is better to be overlubricated rather than underlubricated). As in the previous technique, this stroke can cause discomfort over whisker stubble, so stroke lightly over this area without lubricant. If the discomfort is too severe, avoid this application entirely.

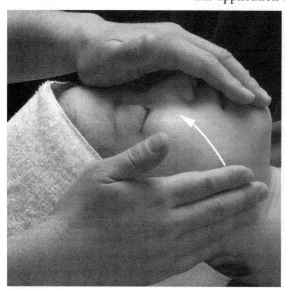

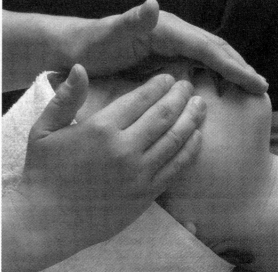

1 You can turn the head 45° to the left for better access to the right cheek. Work on one side of the face at a time. Place the heel of your left hand lightly on the forehead to stabilize the head, then relax the hand so it covers the front of the face. Position your right hand as shown in Example #6.

2 With your right hand, begin the stroke of Example #6. As the fingertips reach the cheekbone, place the pads of the fingers of your left hand on the center of the chin to initiate the alternating stroke. Simultaneously move the right hand slightly away from the face to make room for the left-hand stroke.

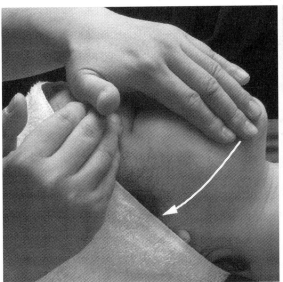 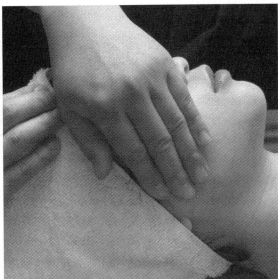

3 The alternating stroke uses only the pads of the first phalanges—the fingertips do not touch the face. Stroke lightly along the crest of the jawbone from the chin to the side of the earlobe. Pivot the hand from its light anchor on the forehead, using the movement of the shoulder and elbow to make the stroke.

4 As the left hand finishes stroking at the side of the ear, place the fingers of the right hand back on the middle of the jawbone to repeat the entire procedure. Alternate strokes continuously with both hands three to seven times or longer if desired. Apply strokes to the left cheek, reversing your hands accordingly.

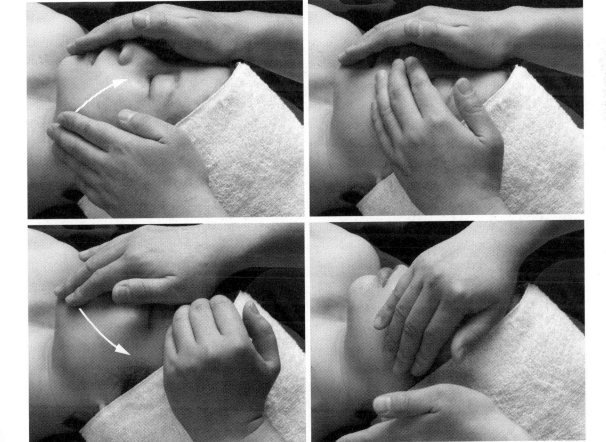

Japanese Facial-Massage Techniques—Example #8

Flip-Stroking on the Jawbone with the Thumb

Japanese name for this technique

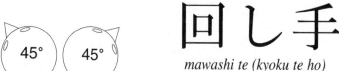

mawashi te (kyoku te ho)

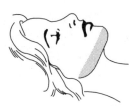

45 Degree Position

The purpose of this technique

Stimulate facial tissue along the jaw

Area of application

Along the jawline

Description

Generous Lubrication

This percussive technique uses a quick, short flip-stroke to stimulate the skin. Do not pinch during the application, and do not let your thumb and index finger touch. When the instructions say "stroke," remember this is also a percussive technique, with quick contact with the skin and a swift takeaway motion providing the "stroke." This is one of the essential fundamental techniques of Japanese facial massage. Practice this technique until you can apply it smoothly on the jaw before trying to apply it on the cheekbone under the eyes (see Example #11).

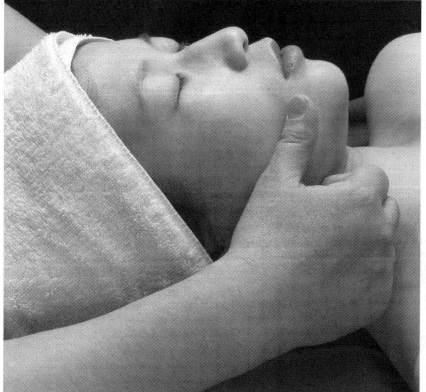

1 With the client's head tilted about 45° to the left, gently place your left hand over the left ear for stabilization. With the right index finger curved in, place the lateral edge of the first two phalanges underneath the jawbone, and place the lateral edge of your thumb on top of the jawbone, as shown. Throughout this application, keep the remaining fingers relaxed and away from the palm.

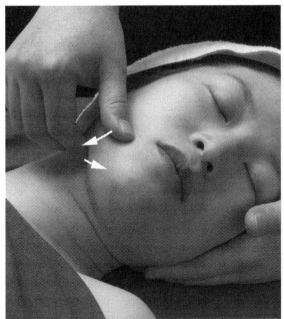

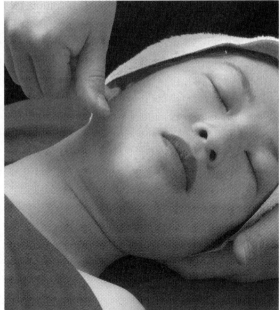

2 The edge of the thumb must be about one half inch to one inch above the edge of the jaw. Quickly stroke away from your body with your thumb, while simultaneously stroking with your index finger by pulling from under the jaw toward you.

3 With this movement, the entire hand jumps up slightly from the jaw, and to avoid pinching, the thumb and index finger must not contact each other on the takeaway. This movement is like a gentle snap, done very quickly and repeated rapidly and continuously.

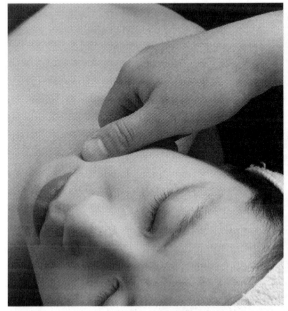

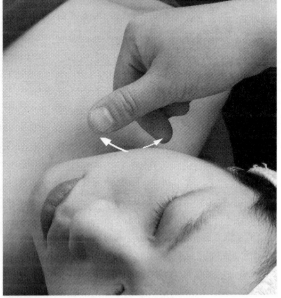

4 This is not a pinching technique: the thumb and index finger are stroking in different directions. Do as much of the work using wrist movements as possible. Use a continuous succession of strokes to move up and down the jaw from chin to ear.

5 Cover all of the jawbone region that your fingertips can easily slide beneath. Run this technique up and down the jaw two or three times or as long as desired. As in the previous technique, it is better to overlubricate than to risk pulling the facial skin.

Japanese Facial-Massage Techniques—Example #9

Two-Finger Walking on the Cheeks

Japanese name for this technique

二指軽擦法

ni shi kei satsu ho

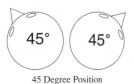

45 Degree Position

The purpose of this technique

Stabilize the region that is receiving the flip-stroking techniques

Area of application

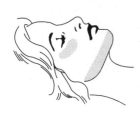

Above the cheekbone and the edge of the jaw

Description

This example is generally used in combination with the flip-stroking techniques (Examples #8 and #11). It is usually done with the left hand since the right hand does the flip-stroking on both sides of the face. Practice this application with the left hand until you are comfortable with it on both sides of the face and have mastered it to the point where you can apply it automatically alongside the flip-stroke.

Generous Lubrication

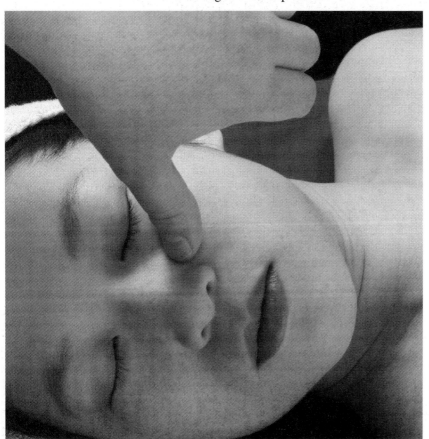

Cheekbone on the Left Side

This technique is explained for the left side of the face, as it is easier to practice with the left hand in this way.

1 To work the left side of the face, tilt the client's head about 45° to the right. Place your left thumb lightly over the cheekbone.

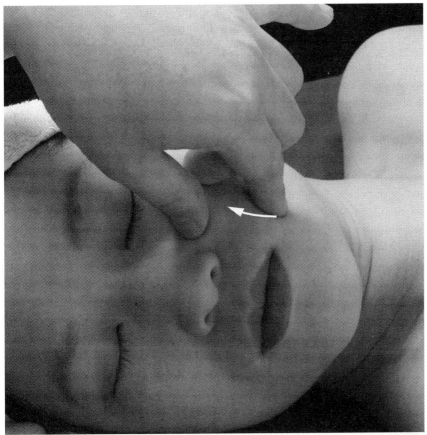

2 Place the index and middle fingers just below the cheek-bone. Apply enough pressure with the thumb to keep your hand stable. Alternate short strokes with the index and middle fingers, pulling them back toward the thumb, as if they were "walking in place."

3 Use enough lubrication for your fingers to slide easily over the surface of the skin. Use only enough pressure to draw the fingertips over the surface of the skin so it does not feel like pinching. It is a very light, short stroke. As you do the technique with your index and middle fingers, gradually shift your hand back and forth, on the thumb, to cover the entire area under the cheekbone (inferior edge of zygomatic bone).

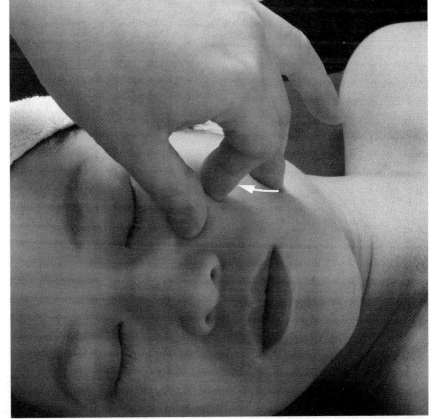

Cheekbone on the Right Side

This is the same technique, still using the left hand, applied to the right side of the face.

4 Tilt the head about 45° to the left. This procedure is identical to Steps 1 through 3, but you must allow the left elbow to raise up high so the hand can be at the proper angle to the face. This slightly awkward position is only be necessary for thirty seconds at most.

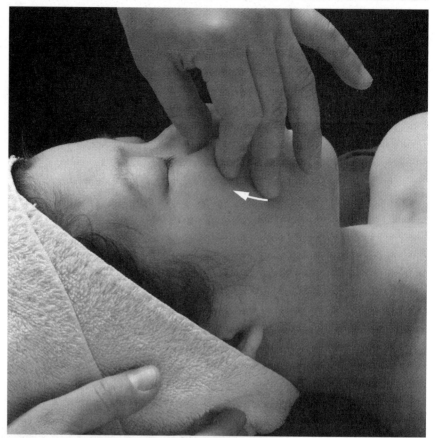

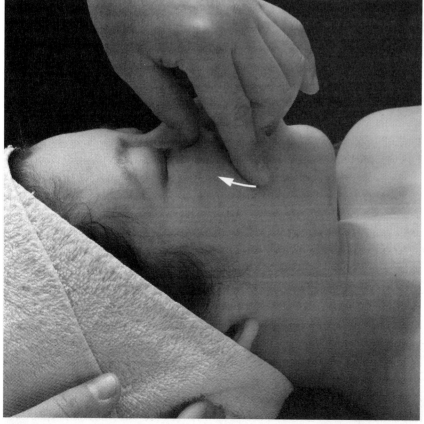

5 Again, keep your thumb over the cheekbone and let it glide over the lower edge as the fingers apply the strokes. The hand does not actually "walk" ahead: the movement of the hand is to the side, away from and back toward the nose (medially and laterally across zygomatic bone).

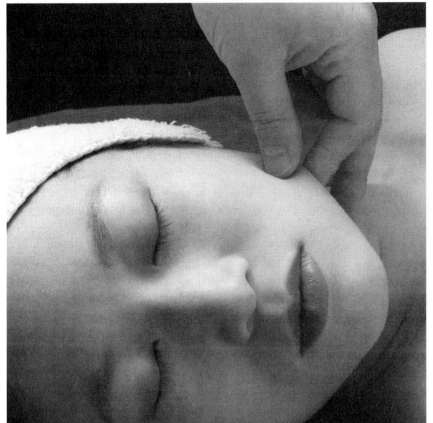

Edge of the Jaw

This is similar to Steps 1 through 3, but it is applied to the edge of the jaw instead of over the cheekbone.

6 Place your left thumb on the superior edge of the jawbone with the tips of the fingers on the inferior edge of the jawbone.

7 Walk across the jawbone with the same strokes used in Step 2. If your client has a beard, you may not need any lubrication; just work slowly. Work up and down the length of the jawbone and then repeat on the right side.

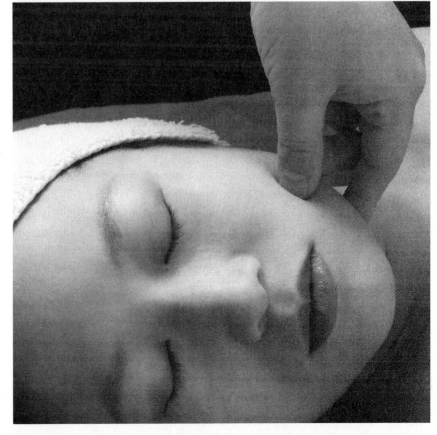

Japanese Facial-Massage Techniques—Example #10

Combination Stroking over the Edge of the Jaw

Japanese name for this technique

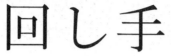

mawashi te (kyoku te ho)

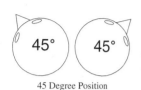

45 Degree Position

The purpose of this technique

Improve the facial tone and appearance along the length of the jawbone by gentle stimulation of the nerves

Area of application

Along the length of jawbone

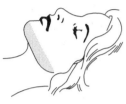

Generous Lubrication

Description

This example is a combination of Examples #8 and #9. Use the finger-walking technique with your index and middle fingers to stabilize the skin surface while the thumb flip-strokes to stimulate the jaw region. When you are able to execute both of these strokes simultaneously, your concentration will be almost entirely on the flip-stroking hand; the finger-walking stroke should require no attention. This example is demonstrated on the left side of the face.

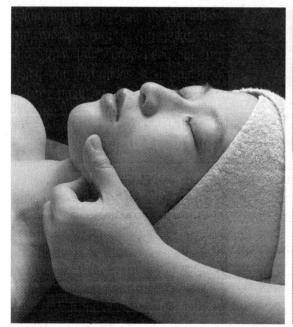

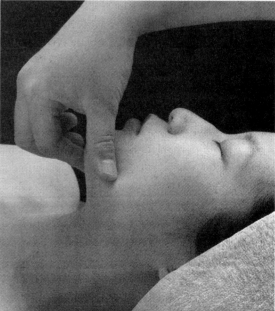

1 This is the proper left-hand position for the finger-walking stroke on the left side of the face (see Example #9). Keep your fingertips underneath the chin and the thumb on the top edge of the jawbone.

2 This is the proper positioning for flip-stroking with the right hand when working on the left side of the face (see Example #8). Place the index fingers under the chin and the thumb on the top edge of the jawbone.

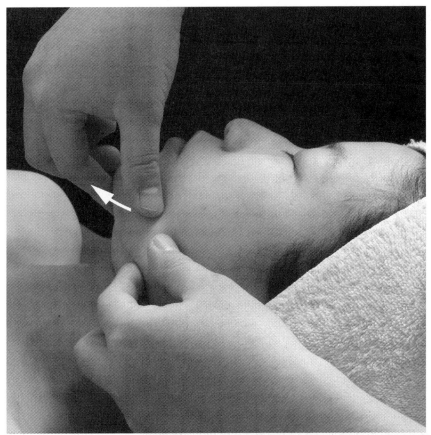

3 This is simply the combination of flip-stroking with the right hand while finger-walking with the left hand. Your thumbs should face each other throughout this movement as the hands trace back and forth across the jawbone. Traverse across the entire length of jawbone two to three times during the cleansing stage and one or two times during the moisturizing stage. Move both hands as a unit, maintaining an inch of separation between your thumbs.

4 Both applications are very light, and there should be absolutely no sensation of pulling on the skin. Again, it is best to overlubricate rather than risk pulling the facial skin due to underlubrication. It is easiest to work both sides of the face with the right hand doing the flip-stroke and the left hand finger-walking. You can reverse these if you wish, but it is not necessary to do so.

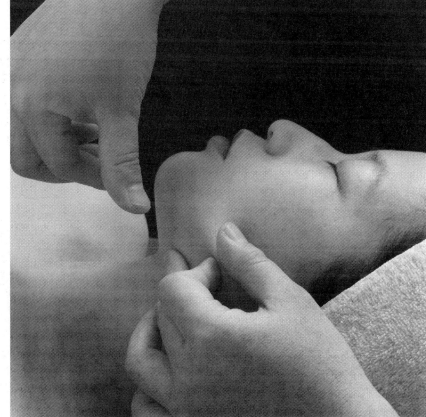

Japanese Facial-Massage Techniques—Example #11

Flip-Stroking on the Top of the Cheekbone

Japanese name for this technique

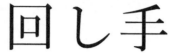

mawashi te (kyoku te ho)

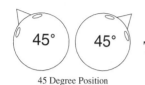

45 Degree Position

The purpose of this technique

Increase circulation and improve appearance by stimulating nerves above cheekbone and around bottom edge of eye

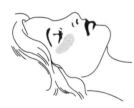

Area of application

Along the superior edge of cheekbone and around bottom edge of eye

Description

Generous Lubrication

This stroke is identical to Example #8, except that it is applied to the top edge of cheekbone. Practice Example #8 until you are very confident with this application before using it on the delicate tissue near the eyes. Use plenty of lubrication to prevent pulling the client's skin.

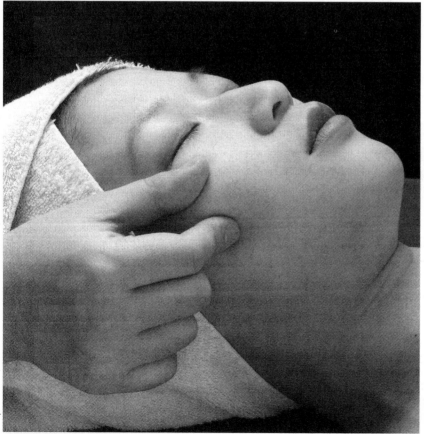

1 Tilt the client's head 45° to the left side and support with the left hand. Gently lay the side of your right thumb along the top edge of the cheekbone. Position your index or middle finger (you can use either) on the inferior edge of the cheekbone. Again, relax your fingers away from your palm, and let the palm maintain a rounded hollow.

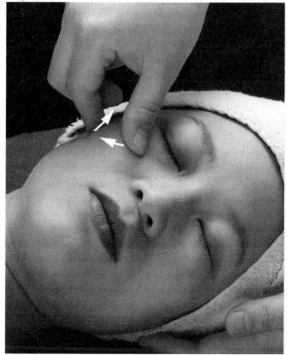 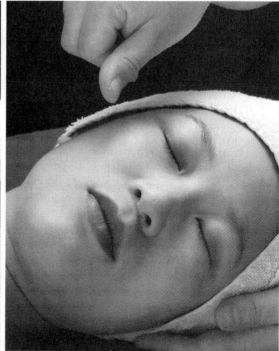

2 This is the same flip-stroke, but be careful when you work around the eyes. The tissue immediately beneath the eyelid is not to be worked directly, so keep clear of the tissue within the first quarter-inch below the lid. The tissue to be worked lies over the cheekbone, particularly the superior edge.

3 The hand jumps up softly as before, but take care near the eyes for the return. Adjust the depth of the stroke by using the lateral edge of the thumb for a light stroke or by increasing the angle of the thumb and using part of the thumbtip for a more penetrating stroke. Cover the length of the upper cheekbone.

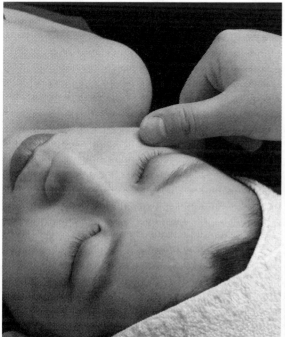 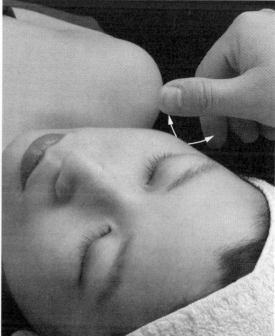

Here is the application as viewed by the practitioner.

Japanese Facial-Massage Techniques—Example #12

Combination Stroking on Top of the Cheekbone

Japanese name for this technique

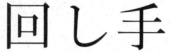

mawashi te (kyoku te ho)

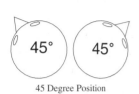

45 Degree Position

The purpose of this technique

Increase circulation and improve appearance by stimulating nerves above cheekbone and around bottom edge of eye

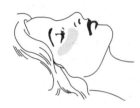

Area of application

Along the superior edge of cheekbone and around the bottom edge of eye

Description

This stroke is identical to Example #10, except it works over the cheek as covered in Examples #9 and #11. Finger walking stabilizes the tissue for the flip-stroke and minimizes pulling of the facial skin. This is one of the core techniques of Japanese facial massage, so practice until you can apply it smoothly and comfortably.

Generous Lubrication

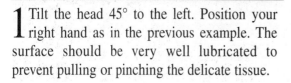

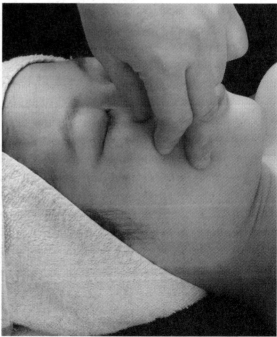

1 Tilt the head 45° to the left. Position your right hand as in the previous example. The surface should be very well lubricated to prevent pulling or pinching the delicate tissue.

2 Place your left hand in the same manner as in Steps 4 and 5 from Example #9.

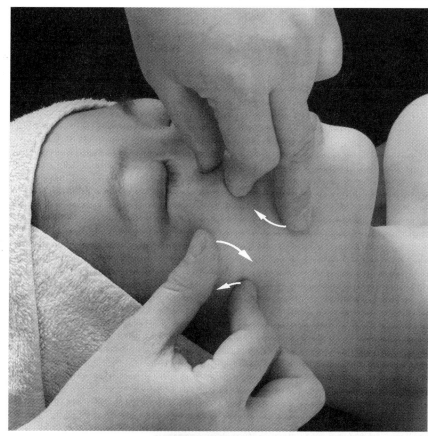

3 Stroke away from the eye with the side of your right thumb while flip-stroking the right index finger in toward your palm. This is the same flipping technique used in Example #11. Use your elbow and wrist to make the flip-stroke, and keep the wrist as free and open as possible. The flip-stroke should not be made by pinching the fingers together.

4 Move your hands as a unit, as in Example #10, but keep only a half-inch distance between the thumbtips. Traverse across the top edge of the cheekbone following the natural contour of the zygomatic bone under the eye. Make three to five passages for the cleansing stage and one to two passages for the moisturizing stage.

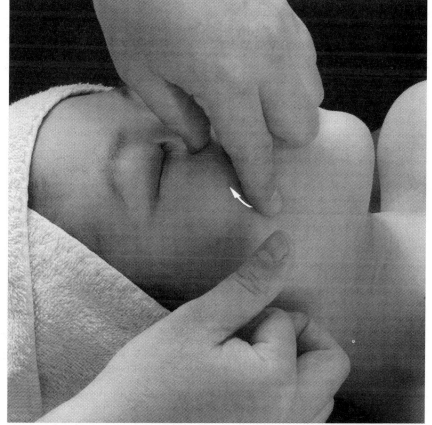

Japanese Facial-Massage Techniques—Example #13

Light Stroking up the Cheek with Two Fingers

Japanese name for this technique

二指軽擦法

(ryo) ni shi kei satsu ho

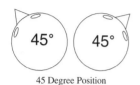

45 Degree Position

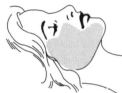

Generous Lubrication

The purpose of this technique

Redistribute the lubrication evenly over skin between techniques

Area of application

Over the entire cheek

Description

This is very similar to Example #7, although this is applied with one or two fingers on each hand and is a much lighter application. This stroke is often used as a bridge between other applications to evenly redistribute the cleanser or moisturizer across the cheek. In general, apply this stroke once or twice in between other techniques.

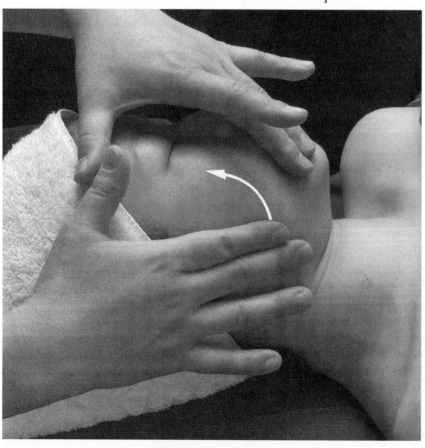

1 Keep the client's head tilted about 45° to the left. Rest the side of each thumb lightly on the temple. The fingers of your left hand should rest against the side of the chin. Place the right index and middle fingers on the right jawbone. Begin stroking over the cheek toward the eye. This stroke can be done with a combination of index and middle fingers, middle and ring fingers, or index or middle finger alone (for a gentle application).

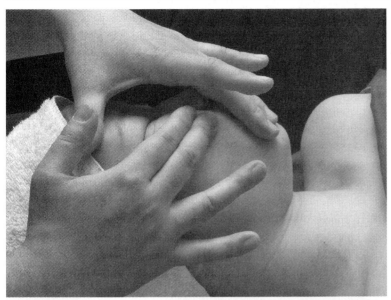

2 The stroke ends at this position over the cheek-bone. As you bring the stroke up the cheek, your palm should rotate toward you, allowing the use of the medial edge of the fingers. Use the entire flat surface of the fingers, instead of the fingertips, for this stroke.

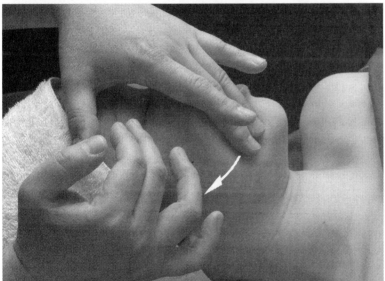

3 As the right hand finishes stroking, begin stroking with the fingers of the left hand. Use this hand to stroke along the jawline up to the front of client's ear. Lift your right hand slightly away from the face to accommodate the passage of the left hand.

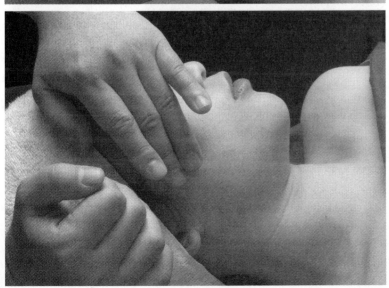

4 As the left fingers finish the stroke, replace the right hand to begin another stroke and continue to stroke alternately with a smooth rhythm of left and right hands. This motion must come from the shoulders and back; it is not simply a finger or hand motion. You can vary the speed and the size of the stroke.

Japanese Facial-Massage Techniques—Example #14

Kneading the Chin with the Thumbs

Japanese name for this technique

拇指頭揉捏法

(ryo) bo shi to ju netsu ho

0°

Center Position

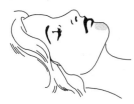

No Lubrication

The purpose of this technique

Increase circulation and relax the muscles of the chin

Area of application

Entire region from base of lip to underside of chin

Description

The first eight techniques in this chapter showed how to apply Japanese facial massage to the sides of the face with the head in the 45° position. The next twelve techniques are mainly applied to the center of the face with the head in the center position. This is a kneading technique, not a stroking technique. This type of kneading is a unique feature of Japanese facial massage, and it is an excellent way to reduce tension of the chin. As with the anma kneading technique, use very little or no lubrication.

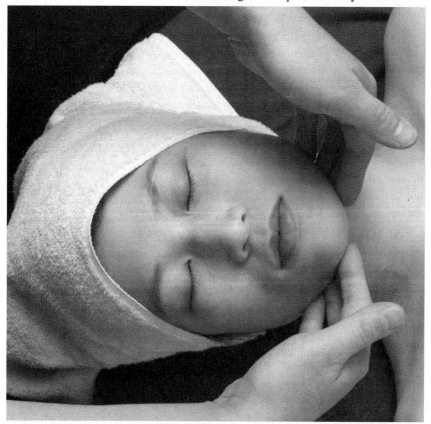

1 Gently move the client's head to the center position. Place the tips of your fingers along the underside of jawbone as shown. Keep your shoulders and arms relaxed.

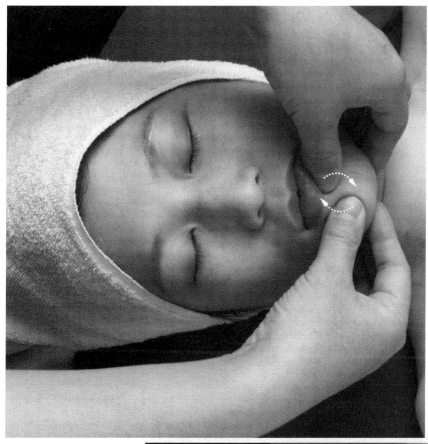

2 Place your thumbs one inch apart with the tips facing each other. With light downward pressure, bring your thumbs inward to create a ridge of skin between them, until they are about one half-inch apart. Knead this ridge and the muscle beneath the thumbs by pressing your thumbtips just past one another, first to one side and then to the other side, in a half-circular rotation.

3 As you knead the chin, move the skin with the thumbs, but do not slide over the skin. Do not bend the thumbs, and do not let the thumbnail contact the skin. Keep you wrists upright, with the thumbs at about 45° to the face. The chin can withstand a good amount of pressure without discomfort. If necessary, bring this motion up and down to cover the entire chin region. Repeat for fifteen to twenty seconds or as long as desired.

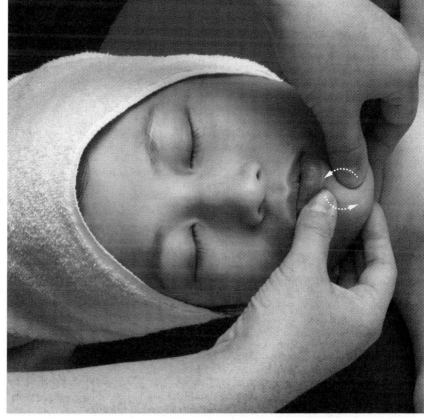

Japanese Facial-Massage Techniques—Example #15

Pressure and Rotation on the Center of the Chin

Japanese names for these techniques

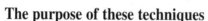

拇指頭圧迫法

bo shi to ap paku ho (Step 2)
bo shi to ju netsu ho (Step 3)

0°

Center Position

The purpose of these techniques

Increase circulation and relax muscles of chin

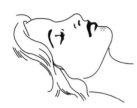

Area of application

Directly on the center of the chin, at *sho sho* (Conception Vessel-24)

Description

No Lubrication

This application is often done in conjunction with the previous application to effectively treat the chin. The chin can generally tolerate strong pressure, although it can be sensitive on some people. Adjust pressure accordingly. Again, no lubrication is necessary for the chin.

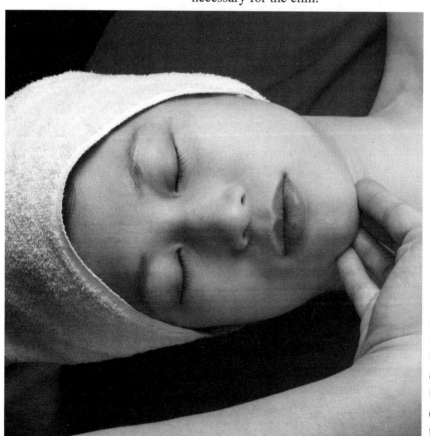

1 Keep the client's head in the center position. To stabilize the application, place the fingertips of three or four fingers under the chin as shown. You can use either hand for this application.

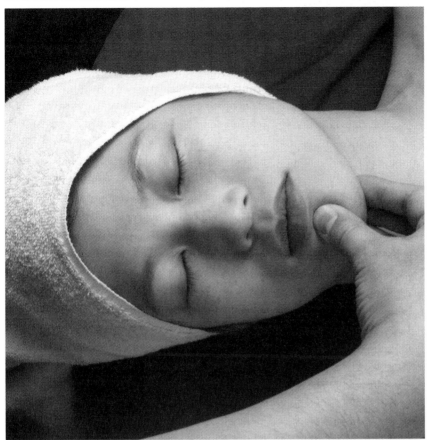

Thumb Pressure

2 Place the tip of your thumb on the *sho sho* (Conception Vessel-24). This *tsubo* is found at the small depression in the center of the chin cleft. Apply pressure for three to five seconds using the thumbpad. Do not let the nail contact the skin. Repeat two or three times.

Thumb Rotation

3 Keep the same hand position used in Step 2. Apply medium pressure, making small rotations. **Do not rotate your thumb from the carpometacarpal joint**: the hand and thumb should rotate as one unit. The rotations should be no larger than a quarter-inch in diameter. Do not slide over the surface of the skin or move the face during the rotation. Apply for five to seven seconds or longer if desired.

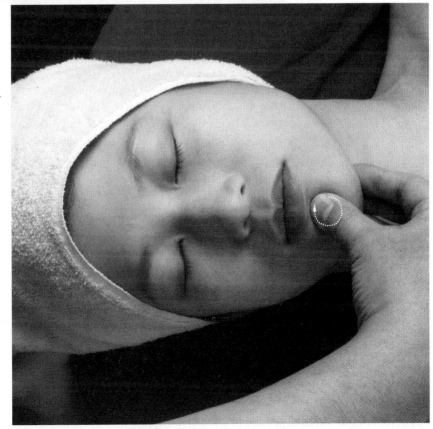

Japanese Facial-Massage Techniques—Example #16

Thumb Pressure on the Lower Face

Japanese name for this technique

拇指頭圧迫法

bo shi to ap paku ho

Center Position

The purpose of this technique

Reduce tension in the chin and jaw, improve appearance, and help prevent wrinkles in lower jaw region.

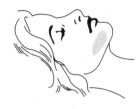

Area of application

On jaw near gumline, approached at sides of chin

Description

No Lubrication

This technique applies pressure to *tsubo* on the jaw. Stimulating these *tsubo* reduces tension and revitalizes the lower face. These acupoints are called *ki ketsu,* which translates to "strange or extraordinary *tsubo*" because they do not belong to specific meridians. *Ki ketsu* points are very important within Japanese facial massage. Here, we use three *ki ketsu* points to stimulate the lower face.

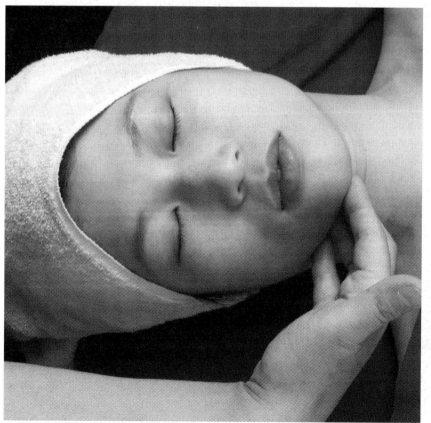

1 With the client's head in the center position, place your fingertips as in Example #15 but slightly out from the center of the chin (lateral), and along the jawbone. Support the left side of head with your left hand.

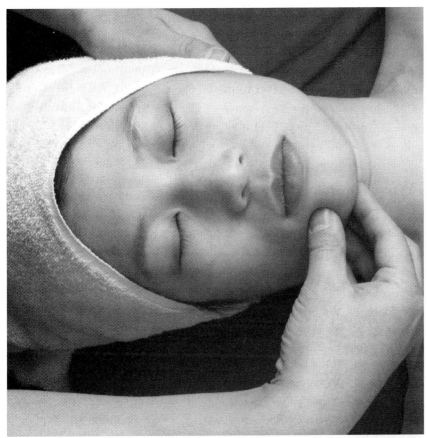

2 Place the tip of your thumb just above the jaw on the side of the chin at *kyo sho sho*. This point is found in a depression at the base of the gum along the jawbone, two thumb-widths lateral from *sho sho* (Conception Vessel-24).

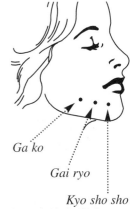

Ga ko

Gai ryo

Kyo sho sho

3 Apply medium pressure toward the gum for three to five seconds, and then move to each of the next two points by finding the depressions one and two thumb-widths from *kyo sho sho*. When each point has been stimulated in turn, come back to *kyo sho sho* and repeat the procedure. After working these points two to three times on one side of the face, repeat the procedure on the other side.

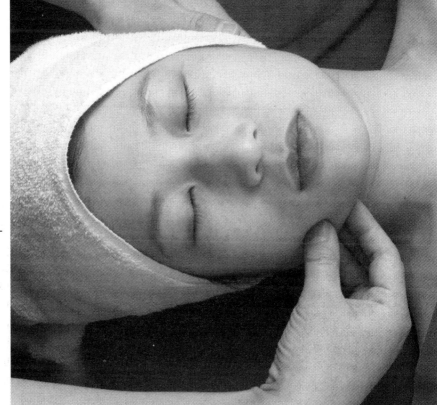

Japanese Facial-Massage Techniques—Example #17

Kneading the Forehead with the Thumbs

Japanese name for this technique

拇指揉捏法

(ryo) bo shi ju netsu ho

0°

Center Position

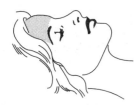

No Lubrication

The purpose of this technique

Increase circulation, improve appearance, and prevent wrinkles on the forehead

Area of application

The entire forehead

Description

This technique is identical to Example #14, except that it is applied on the forehead. This and the next technique are the primary techniques for working on the forehead. Lubrication is not necessary, although you can use some lotion if you choose. You can apply quite a bit of pressure on the forehead without making the client uncomfortable.

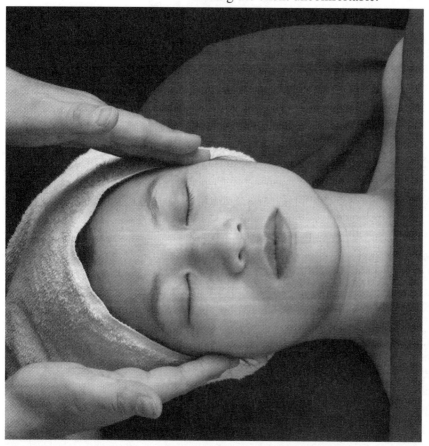

1 With the client's head in the center position, lightly place the tips of your index and middle fingers or your middle and ring fingers just inferior to the temple region to stabilize head and hands. Adjust the placement of the fingertips to accommodate the positioning of your thumbs.

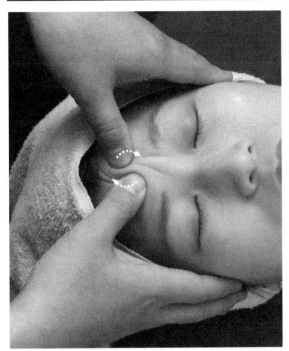

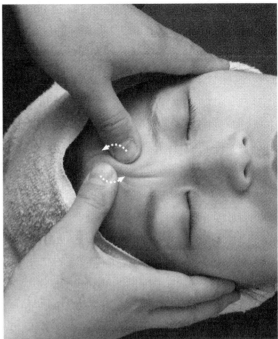

2 Place the thumbs about one thumb-width apart on the forehead near hairline. Begin application by applying firm downward pressure and knead in the same manner as shown in Example #14.

3 The thumbs should knead in opposite directions and gradually move toward the area between the eyebrows. Use enough pressure to keep the thumbs from sliding over the skin.

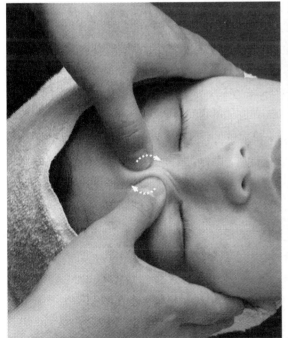

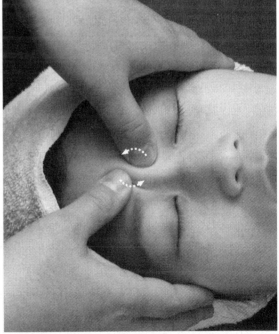

4 You can apply slightly greater pressure between the eyebrows. Return to the hairline, moving one thumb-width to the side, and repeat the procedure.

5 It is easier to work from the hairline toward the eyebrows. Work in vertical sections, one thumb-width across, until you have covered the forehead.

Stroking on the Forehead with the Palms

Japanese name for this technique

0°

Center Position

拇指球軽擦法

(ryo) bo shi kyu kei satsu ho

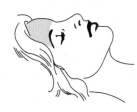

Minimal Lubrication

The purpose of this technique

Clear toxins from the lymphatic system after kneading application

Area of application

On the entire forehead

Description

This is the second of the two most common techniques for massaging the forehead. The previous kneading application tends to bring toxins to the surface, and this stroke—a much lighter application—provides good lymphatic drainage to clear these toxins from the forehead. This stroke generally follows the previous application. Slight lubrication is required for this technique.

This example is very similar to Example #42 (explained in Chapter 10), except in this technique the lower palms and the heels of the hands and are used, rather than the thumbs. In fact, both Examples #18 and #42 are often combined together seamlessly in actual practice.

This technique can be used at any point during the treatment, although I use it as a finishing touch.

You must maintain a minimal amount of lubrication so you neither stretch nor pull the skin.

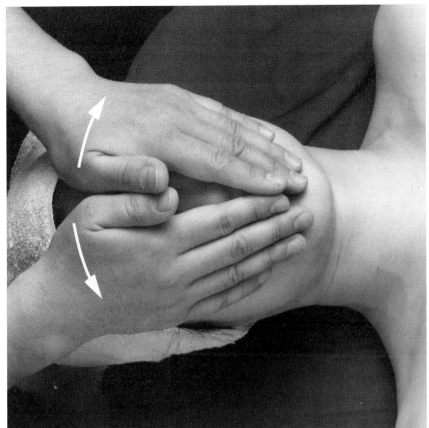

1 Gently place the tips of your middle and ring fingers just above the client's jaw on either side of the chin. Place the balls of the thumbs (thenar) side by side on the center of the forehead. Apply extremely light pressure, so you are barely touching the surface of the fore-head, and slowly slide the balls of the thumbs away from each other toward the temple region. Do not slide the middle and ring fingers with the stroke—use the fingers as a pivot point for the movement.

2 Finish stroking over the temple region. Gently release your hands and repeat two to three times. Use just enough pressure to contact the skin, yet the sides of the thumbs should be in full contact to fit the contour of the forehead. Repeat three to five times.

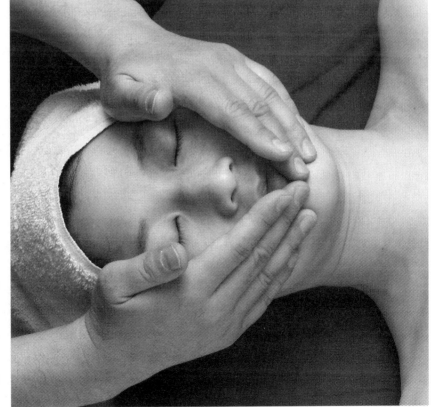

Japanese Facial-Massage Techniques—Example #19

Light Percussion on the Face with Four Fingers

Japanese names for these techniques

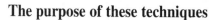

四指叩打法

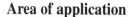

shi shi ko da ho (Steps 1 through 2)
shi shi to ko da ho (Steps 3 through 6)

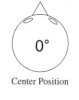

0°

Center Position

The purpose of these techniques

Increase facial circulation by stimulating nerves

Area of application

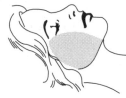

The entire cheek

Description

No Lubrication

Gentle percussion techniques stimulate facial nerves. This improves circulation, which is essential to improve facial tone, prevent wrinkles, and repair facial tissues. Percussion here must be applied from within one inch of the surface of the skin. As in all percussion, the fingers should be kept loose as you tap the area, or the client will feel discomfort. Percussion can be applied on both sides of the face at the same time it can alternate. The techniques should be applied rhythmically and smoothly. Practice on yourself to get the feel of the technique and the pressure. No lubrication is necessary.

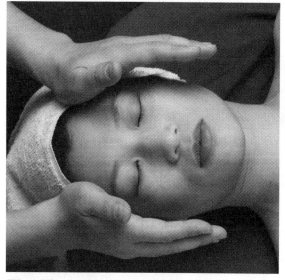

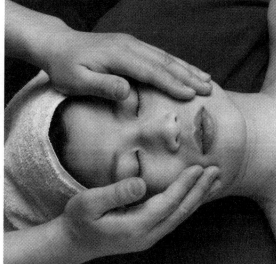

Flat Fingers

1 Place the heels of your hands lightly above the temple region. Gently tap the cheeks with loosely flattened fingers.

2 Continue a soft percussive tap for ten to twenty seconds. You can either apply to one side of the face at a time or both sides at once.

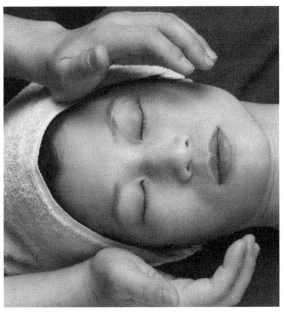
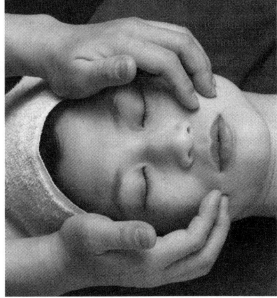

Fingertips Together

3 With heels of your hands resting lightly on the client's head, curl the fingers slightly and tap loosely with the fingertips, moving from the wrists.

4 This technique covers small sections of tissue at a time. Move your hand as a unit to cover the cheek thoroughly. You can apply this technique to the temple region if desired.

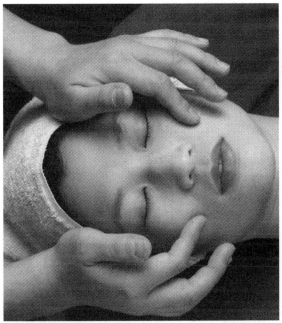
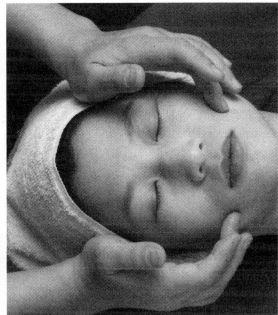

Separate Fingertips

5 In this variation, you move only the fingers and not the wrist. The fingers should tap the face, one after another, as in playing the piano or typing. Move to cover the entire cheek.

6 This is the lightest of all three techniques: be sure your fingers are loose. Smooth, quick finger movements require practice.

Japanese Facial-Massage Techniques—Example #20
Finger Stroking on the Side of the Nose

Japanese name for this technique

Center Position

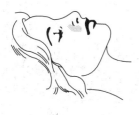

指頭軽擦法

shi to kei satsu ho

The purpose of this technique

Remove dirt and oil from crease along nostrils

Area of application

Around the lateral crease of nostrils

Minimal Lubrication

Description

The lateral creases of the nostril often collect facial dirt and oil. This technique is generally used during the cleansing stage to remove unwanted material from the skin. You may stroke once or twice in this area during the moisturizing stage but this technique should be primarily used during the cleansing stage. Make sure that your nails do not touch the facial tissue.

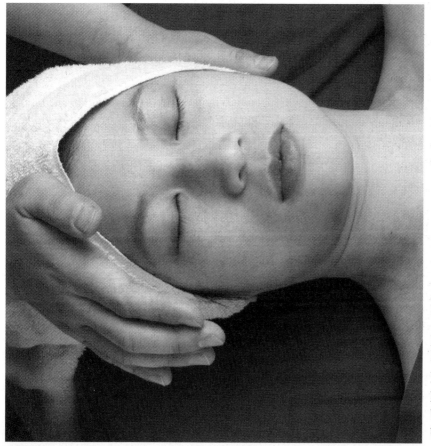

1 With the client's head in the center position, support the left side of head with your left hand. Gently place the heel of your thumb on the forehead to stabilize your hand.

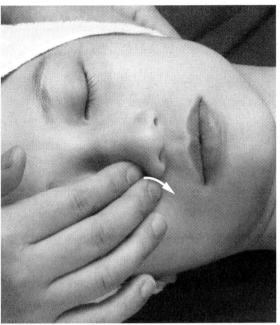

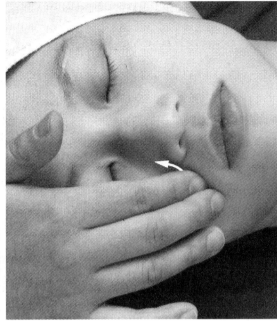

Stroking the Crease of the Nose

2 Curl your fingers and place the tips of your index and middle fingers along the side of the nose. Stroke lightly down the side of the nose and along the nasolabial groove.

3 Continue the stroke until your fingers cannot extend further, and stroke back to the starting position. Repeat four to five times or longer depending on the amount of oil on the face.

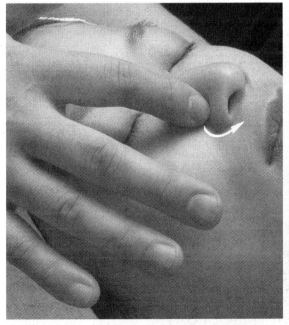

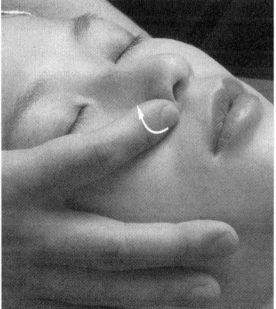

Stroking the Edge of the Nose (Nares)

4 Place the tip of your index finger in the crease of the nose. Stroke gently down the crease with your hand away from the head. Do not contact the face with your fingernails.

5 Rotate your finger just enough to keep the tip pressed into the crease. Return the stroke along the same path. Repeat four to five times or longer if necessary.

Japanese Facial-Massage Techniques—Example #21

Circular Stroking on the Side of the Nose

Japanese name for this technique

Center Position

二指軽擦法

(ryo) ni shi kei satsu ho

The purpose of this technique

Increase circulation around nose and sinus openings

Area of application

On the side of the nose and cheeks between eye and nose

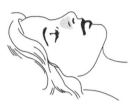

Description

Examples #20 through #22 are geared primarily to the cleansing stage to remove dirt and excessive oil from the region around the nose. This region is one of the oiliest areas of the face, and these three techniques work together to clean these tissues gently and thoroughly. When you work the side of the nose, monitor your pressure so you do not even momentarily block respiration in the nasal passages.

Minimal Lubrication

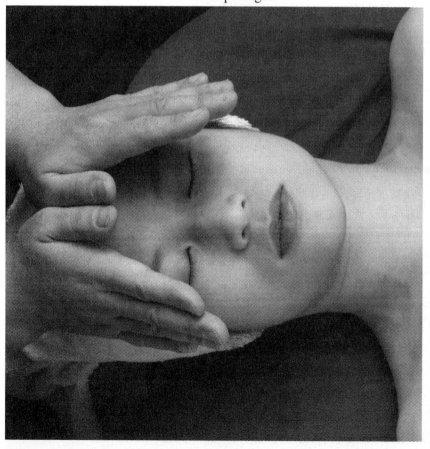

1 With the client's head in the center position, gently place the heels of your hands next to each other on the forehead. Your palms should cup the eyebrows so the fingertips can reach the nose.

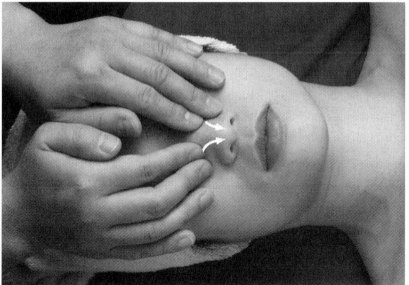

2 Place the tips of the index and middle fingers at the sides of nose, slightly overlapping one another. Begin stroking at the side of the nose, and work the fingertips up across the nostrils to the tip of the nose. Follow the contour of the nose by allowing your palms to rotate inward so index and middle fingers face one another at the tip of nose.

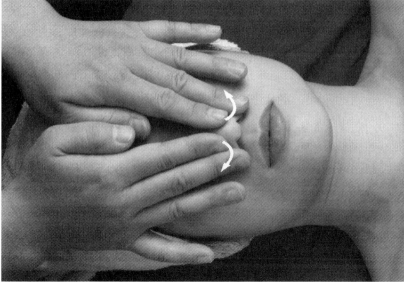

3 Stroke in a circle following the contours down the sides of the nostrils. When you have stroked down the nostrils and are off of the nose entirely, allow your hands to flatten against the cheeks.

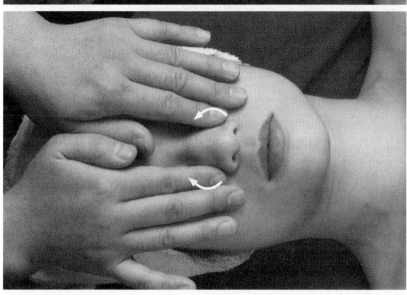

4 Continue your stroke by circling laterally from the nose along the bordering medial cheek tissue back in the direction of the starting position. Maintain a continuous circular motion, using minimum lubrication to glide over the skin. Complete five to seven circular strokes or more if desired.

Japanese Facial-Massage Techniques—Example #22

Stroking on the Nose

Japanese name for this technique

三指軽擦法

(ryo) san shi kei satsu ho

0°

Center Position

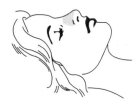

Minimal Lubrication

The purpose of this technique

Remove excess oil from the nose during cleansing stage and redistribute moisturizer during the moisturizing stage

Area of application

On the top and sides of the nose

Description

The tip of the nose often collects excess amounts of oil, so spend extra time here during the cleansing stage. Use light pressure with a fair amount of cleanser. During the moisturizing stage, one or two strokes is sufficient. As in the previous example, avoid applying this technique with too much pressure or too slowly, so you do not block the client's air flow.

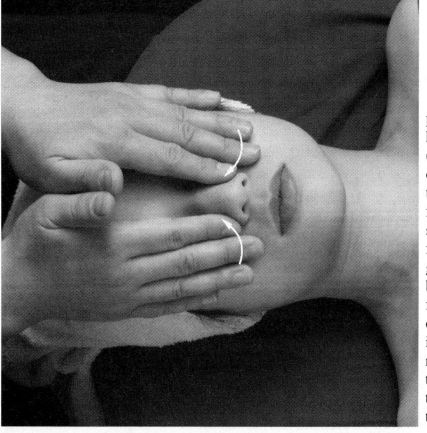

1 With the client's head in the center position, place the heels of both thumbs (thenar surface) lightly on the forehead. Place the fingerpads of the first phalanges to the sides of the nose, and flatten out your fingers. Begin the stroke by drawing your index fingers up the side of nose. Use only the index, middle, and ring fingers for this technique, and keep them straight and together as you stroke.

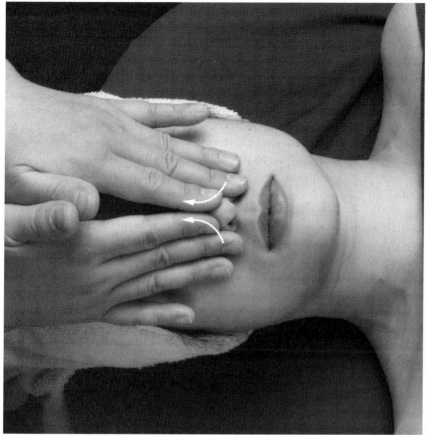

2 Immediately follow your index fingers with the middle and ring fingers. Each finger strokes the nose in turn as it glides towards the tip. As you stroke, let your hands gradually merge until they are facing one another, and the palms are no longer touching the client's forehead.

3 The fingers of both hands should meet at the top of the client's nose as such: index to index, middle to middle, and ring to ring. The stroke is complete when the ring fingers meet and the hand is no longer touching the nose. Repeat three to five times or as desired, depending on the amount of oil on the client's face.

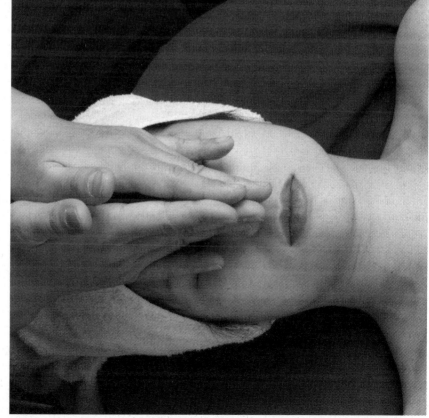

Japanese Facial-Massage Techniques—Example #23

Stroking the Lips

Japanese names for these technique

拇指軽擦法

bo shi kei satsu ho (upper lip)
shi to kei satsu ho (lower lip)
ni shi kei satsu ho (both lips)

Center Position

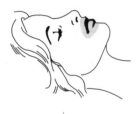

Minimal Lubrication

The purpose of these techniques

Improve appearance around lips

Area of application

On tissue above and below lips

Description

This example demonstrates a technique for working the tissue just above and below the lips. The stroke covers only one side of the face at a time; the practitioner works each side of the face separately. These techniques should be done lightly and smoothly on the facial skin an inch above and below the lips and not touching the mucous membrane (the actual lip tissue).

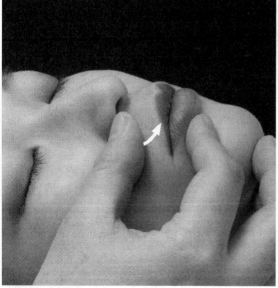

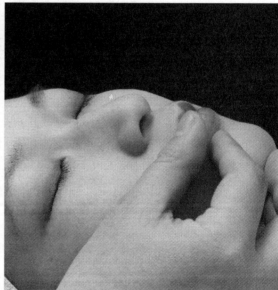

Upper Lip

1 Begin with the head in the center position. Place your index finger at the edge of lower lip to stabilize both your hand and the client's mouth. Place the side of your thumb just below the nostril and stroke toward your index finger.

2 End the stroke at the top of the upper lip. Repeat the stroke several times while moving across the region medially and laterally to cover the entire area above lip.

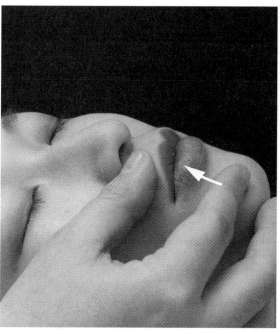

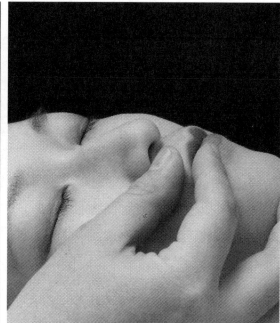

Lower Lip

3 Place your thumb beneath the nostril to stabilize both hand and mouth. The side of your index finger should be half an inch beneath the lower lip. Stroke toward your thumb.

4 End the stroke at the top of the lower lip. Repeat the stroke several times while moving across region medially and laterally to cover the entire area below lip.

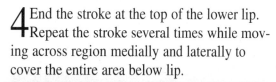

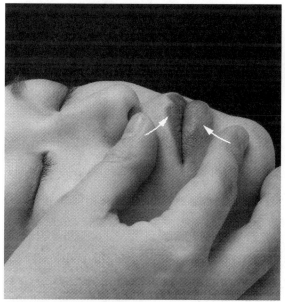

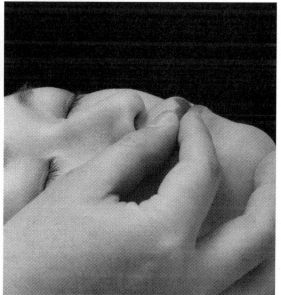

Both Lips Together

5 This is a combination of Steps 1 through 4 and strokes both upper and the lower lips at the same time. This feels like you are trying to pick the lips up, but be careful not to pinch.

6 At the end of the stroke, your index finger and thumb should be touching each other but not touching the lips. Repeat on the left side of the lips using your left thumb and index finger.

Japanese Facial-Massage Techniques—Example #24

Stroking in Front of the Ear

Japanese names for these techniques

拇指軽擦法

bo shi kei satsu ho (Steps 1 through 2)
shi to kei satsu ho (Steps 3 through 4)

0°

Center Position

The purpose of this technique

Improve appearance of side of face in front of ear

Area of application

In front of the ear

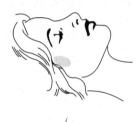

Minimal Lubrication

Descriptions

These techniques work around the front of the ears. Often facial massage leaves this region untouched. By being near the jaw, this area collects much muscle and joint tension, and there are many meridians that gather just in front of the ear. For these reasons, massage in this area can be very beneficial. If you need better access, tilt the client's head as needed.

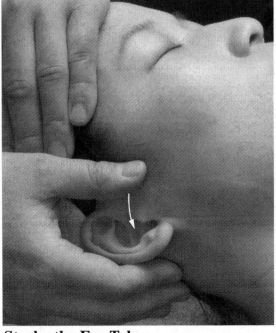

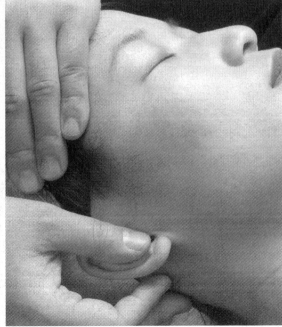

Stroke the Ear Tab

1 With the client's head centered, support the forehead with the palm of your left hand. Place the side of your right thumb in front of ear tab. Stroke gently toward the ear.

2 Stroke toward the ear canal until you pass just onto the ear tab. Do not allow lubricant to enter the ear. Repeat five times on each side.

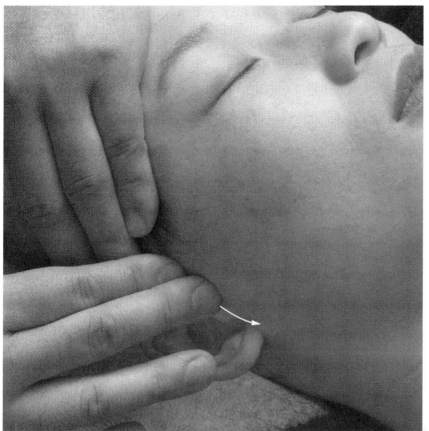

Stroke by the Ear

3 Place your right index finger at the top attachment of the ear and your middle finger in front of it. Stroke with your middle finger, away from the index finger, while your index finger lightly anchors the skin. Use light to medium pressure, and move the finger by bringing the back of your hand forward. Do not let the fingernails touch the client's facial tissue.

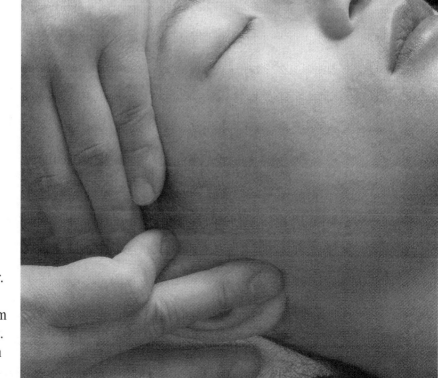

4 Stroke until your middle finger reaches the bottom attachment of the ear. Your index finger should not move from the upper attachment. Repeat three times in front of both ears.

Japanese Facial-Massage Techniques—Example #25

Circular Stroking around the Eyes

Japanese name for this technique

二指頭軽擦法

(ryo) ni shi to kei satsu ho

0°

Center Position

The purpose of this technique

Improve appearance around the eyes

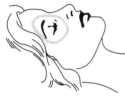

Area of application

Around the eyes and the forehead, including the region above eyebrows

Description

Generous Lubrication

Although this is the last example, it is not necessarily the last technique performed during Japanese facial massage. This technique uses light circular strokes around the eye. It is more commonly used during the moisturizing stage, although it can also be used during the cleansing stage. Use enough lubricant for a smooth application.

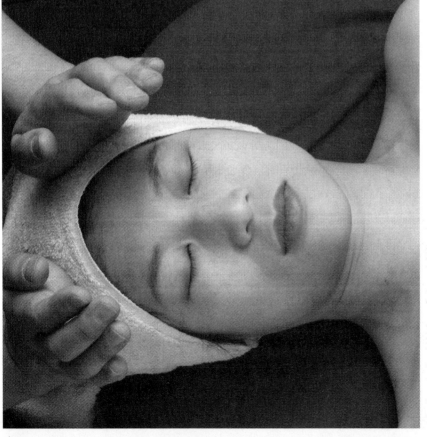

1 With the client's head in the center position, gently rest the heels of your hands above the forehead. The final placement of the heels of the hands may need adjusting according to what is most comfortable and convenient for the application.

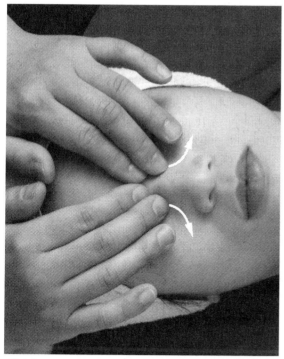

2 Place the tips of your index and middle fingers together at top of nose. Begin stroking down along the sides of the nose.

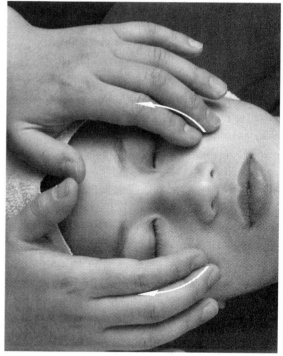

3 Flare outward from the nose and stroke across the cheekbones. Continue stroking toward the temples in a circular motion.

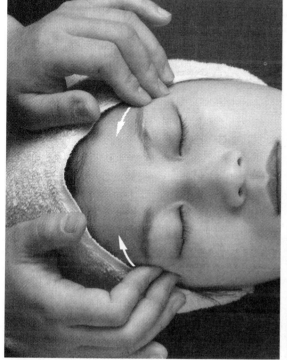

4 As you pass over the temple region, bring the stroke over the eyebrows to the center of forehead. Stroke smoothly using light, even pressure.

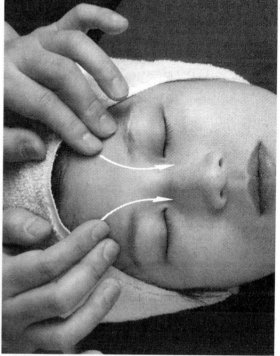

5 Continue the stroke between the eyebrows and down to the top of nose. Each cycle should take two or three seconds; repeat five to seven times or longer if desired.

Chapter Nine
ENERGIZING TECHNIQUES

This chapter introduces the energizing techniques of Japanese facial massage. Energizing techniques are not only unique to Japanese facial massage, they are the very core of Japanese facial-massage treatment. They are also a very effective means to vitalize the face by increasing facial *ki* (life energy or life force).

Generally, Japanese facial massage is comprised of three stages: cleansing, moisturizing, and energizing. Each stage has a unique and important role, and combining the three gives the maximum benefit. Massage techniques in the cleansing and moisturizing stages generally focus on improving circulation and reducing muscle tension. The energizing stage focuses on stimulating the *keiraku* (meridians) and *tsubo* (acupoints or acupuncture points) to increase the facial *ki* flow.

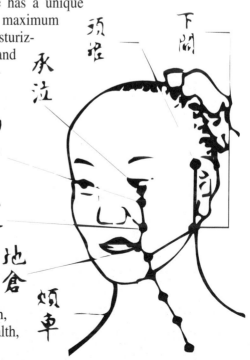

The medical tradition concerning *keiraku* and *tsubo* has been flourishing for over 5,000 years after having originated in ancient China. Japanese facial massage integrates these concepts beautifully, maximizing the benefits of facial massage.

Proper *ki* flow in the face is closely connected to balanced physical and psychological health. As I explained earlier, beauty comes from optimal health, and by balancing the physical and psychological health, it helps to reflect internal balance of the entire body.

Energizing Stages

The benefits of Japanese facial massage far exceed those of regular facial massage. The face interconnects the points of the meridians. Acupuncture is a technique commonly used in giving a face-lift by inserting needles into facial *tsubo*. However, superior effects may be obtained with pressure to *tsubo*. Finger pressure is a more safe and gentle method, and combined with facial-massage techniques, is more effective than acupuncture alone.

The energizing stage consists of two main types of applications. One is the application of pressure directly on the *tsubo*. The other is stroking the meridians. Applying pressure to *tsubo* stimulates certain nerves in the body to improve the appearance of facial tissue as well as improving circulation of body fluids. It is possible to treat certain common ailments through *tsubo*. A meridian is a flow of liquid which carries bioelectricity (*ki*) throughout the body. The movement of bioelectricity through the meridian channels creates a biomagnetic field and polarizes the body. Since twelve internal organs simultaneously create *ki* for the entire body, slight fluctuations occur continuously in the overall harmony of the *ki* flow. When this balance is disturbed beyond a certain point, illness results. One way of rebalancing the *ki* flow is to stroke the meridians.

> **NOTE**
>
> I have in some instances capitalized the names of particular internal organs, and here I am referring to the organ as it is referred to in traditional Northeast Asian medical terminology, which differs from Western medical terminology. If the name of the organ is in lowercase, I am referring to the organ as it is conventionally referred to in Western medicine.

At the professional level of treatment, the practitioner must examine the condition of each meridian and must stroke according to the particular condition of each corresponding organ to help improve the facial condition as well as overall health. For example, if the Small Intestine is *kyo* (depleted), and the Bladder is *jitsu* (excessive), a very slow, gentle stroke along the Small Intestine Meridian in the direction of the *ki* flow (as described in Example #31) and a slightly quicker, heavier stroke of the Bladder Meridian against the *ki* flow (reversing the procedure of Example #33) helps balance the *ki* throughout the face and body. Because I am not explaining Japanese facial diagnosis in this book, it is best for the beginning student to follow the *ki* flow as described (although going against the *ki* flow will not do any harm), which improves the *ki* flow and still produce a nice face-lift effect without any risk.

Keiraku and *tsubo* may look complex when observed together, but by taking one meridian and one point at a time, it is a more simple system to learn. Each individual meridian, as well as each *tsubo*, has very unique characteristics. Before explaining the application of pressure to *tsubo* and methods of stroking certain meridians, I introduce the important concepts of *ki*, *keiraku*, and *tsubo*, and their orientations on the face.

Ki

Ki (pronounced "kee") is the Japanese spelling of Chinese *qi* (pronounced "chee") and means "life-force energy." *Ki* is intricately connected to daily life in Japan. For example, people ask, "How is your *ki* today?" instead of "How are you?" Disease is described as "illness of *ki*" (*byo ki*). In the West, there is no corresponding concept for this sense of integrated being. In my experience, Westerners have great difficulty understanding *ki* because it cannot be explained intellectually. *Ki* is not a revolutionary concept or anything exotic; it is simply the energy that supports the functions of life. According to traditional Taoist theory, there are three types of *ki* energy which affect everything in the universe: *ten ki*, *ji ki*, and *jin ki*.

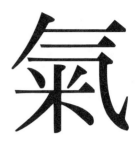

Ki—Universal Energy

1. *Ten Ki* 天気

Ten means "heaven or sky." *Ten ki* comes from everything above ground level. In modern times, it has come to mean weather, because weather is governed by *ten ki*. This is the strongest of all forms of *ki* and affects the other types of *ki*, although it cannot be affected by the other two types of *ki* in return. The condition of the sun, moon, sky, clouds, humidity, and other aspects of weather affect people as well as *ji ki*. Notice how depressed some people become after several cloudy, overcast days—the quality of the *ki* in weather affects humans. It is easy to see how *ten ki* affects *ji ki* in the natural world: insufficient rain (*ten ki*) causes drought (*ji ki*); too much rain (*ten ki*) causes flooding (*ji ki*).

2. *Ji Ki* 地気

Ji means "ground," and *ji ki* comes from the ground. It is *ki* energy from the earth and controls such things as soil, earthquakes, minerals, groundwater, and heat from the earth's core. *Ji ki* is responsible for everything on or in the ground. The condition of *ji ki* is affected by *ten ki*, but not by *jin ki*. Conversely, *ji ki* affects *jin ki* but not *ten ki*. For example, an earthquake affects people but has no direct discernible effect on the weather.

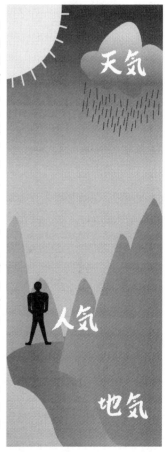

3. *Jin Ki* 人気

Jin ki is human *ki* or the life energy of humans. *Jin ki* has no effect on *ten ki* or *ji ki*, but is affected by both of them. Therefore, the condition of the environment and nature are very important to human life. One must understand the relationships among *ten ki*, *ji ki,* and *jin ki*.

In East Asian medicine, *ki* or "internal *ki*" always refers to *jin ki*. All *ki* is connected to *jin ki*, which means *jin ki* is a part of universal *ki*. It is known that men are more closely connected to *ten ki* (heaven *ki*) and women to *ji ki* (ground *ki*).

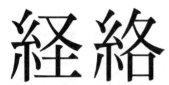

Keiraku
Meridian System

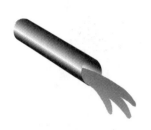

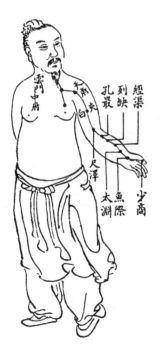

**Meridian illustration
from about 600 B.C.**

Keiraku

Keiraku (commonly translated as "meridian system") are the channels or pathways for *ki* energy. *Keiraku* is traditionally used in anma because it co-evolved with other forms of traditional Northeast Asian medicine. *Keiraku* are liquid vessels with a diameter of twenty to fifty millimicrons. They are pathways for a clear, transparent liquid (*toeki*) and work much like a nerve. Over the last two centuries, the use of the *keiraku* system with anma became less common. One major reason is because at that time anma had become primarily a job for blind people deprived of education. The *keiraku* system is not an easy system to master. It has always been an area of advanced study for experienced therapists.

The *keiraku* (*ching-lo* in Chinese) system consists of a total of 100 meridians and connections. The *keiraku* has a *kei* system and a *raku* system. The *kei* system consists of thirty-two meridian vessels: twelve standard *kei* meridians connected from internal organs, twelve branch meridians ,and eight vessels. The remaining sixty-eight vessels compose the *raku* system and its connections.

The twelve standard *kei* meridians are:

1)	*Hai kei*	Lung Meridian
2)	*Dai cho kei*	Large Intestine Meridian
3)	*I kei*	Stomach Meridian
4)	*Hi kei*	Spleen Meridian
5)	*Shin kei*	Heart Meridian
6)	*Sho cho kei*	Small Intestine Meridian
7)	*Bo ko kei*	Bladder Meridian
8)	*Jin kei*	Kidney Meridian
9)	*Shin po kei*	*Shin Po* Meridian
10)	*San sho kei*	*San Sho* Meridian
11)	*Tan kei*	Gall Bladder Meridian
12)	*Kan kei*	Liver Meridian

The twelve *kei* meridians are connected to each other in the order listed above and form two bilaterally symmetric loops on either side of the body. It takes exactly twenty-four hours for *ki* to cycle through the twelve meridians.

The two vessels divide the body in different directions to balance the meridians. The two vessels which travel along the median line on the front and the back are the two most often used for treatment.

13)	*Nin myaku*	Conception Vessel
14)	*Toku myaku*	Governing Vessel

The combination of the eight vessels and twelve standard *kei* meridians is commonly called the "fourteen meridians on the body." These are most commonly used for diagnosis and treatment in traditional Japanese medicine.

Kyo (depleted) and *Jitsu* (excessive)

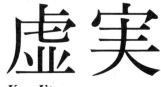

Kyo Jitsu—
Depleted and Excessive

Kyo and *jitsu* are terms used to describe the condition of the *ki* flow in each meridian. The common English translation of *kyo* is "depleted," while *jitsu* is "excessive." In Chinese, they are pronounced as *hsu* (*kyo*) and *hsih* (*jitsu*). Traditional Northeast Asian medicine does not name diseases or illness in the same way Western medicine does. The nature of medicine is also different. Traditional Northeast Asian medicine uses descriptions such as Lung *kyo* and Spleen *jitsu* to name an illness or condition. In Western medicine, medical professionals wait for clear symptoms before diagnosing. In traditional Northeast Asian medicine, conditions are diagnosed long before symptoms develop.

Kyo and *jitsu* describe the stagnation of *ki*. When the term "stagnation" is used, it refers to either too little or too much *ki* flow. Too much *ki* flow does not necessarily mean it is better—it can be just as damaging and can create physical and psychological problems just as too little *ki* flow can.

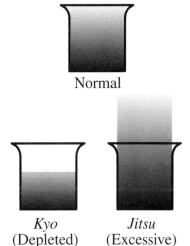

Normal

Kyo
(Depleted)

Jitsu
(Excessive)

Although beginners should be able to determine whether a meridian is regular or irregular, determining *kyo* or *jitsu* is generally thought to be one of the most difficult skills to master in traditional Northeast Asian medicine. Do not be discouraged. It takes much practice to determine whether a condition is *kyo* or *jitsu*, but it is essential to practice and develop the skills to make an accurate diagnosis.

Kyo, the condition of depletion, translates as "lies," "untruths," or "superficial." *Kyo* is a condition of stagnant *ki* flow. The flow is disturbed because not enough energy is flowing through the meridian. *Kyo* symptoms are generally not obvious; they are often hidden and must be sought. An informed diagnosis is generally necessary to discover *kyo* symptoms.

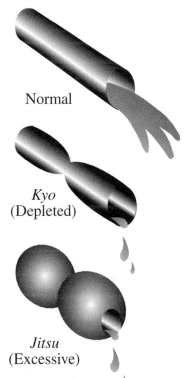

Normal

Kyo
(Depleted)

Jitsu
(Excessive)

Jitsu, the condition of excess, translates as "real," "exists," or "truths." *Jitsu* is the condition in which too much energy flows through the meridian. *Jitsu* symptoms are usually more obvious than *kyo* symptoms and are often found by simply listening to your client's complaints. These would include things such as heat, pain, aches, or other obvious ailments.

Ho and *sha* are other terms used in anma and traditional Japanese medicine. *Ho* is a Japanese name for "tonification" or "supporting." In the context of Northeast Asian medicine, it means to tonify or raise the *kyo* (depleted) condition. *Sha* is the Japanese name for "throwing away" or "taking out." In the context of traditional Japanese medicine, *sha* has come to mean sedation or quieting a condition that is *jitsu* (excess).

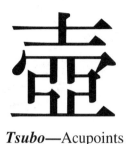

Tsubo—Acupoints

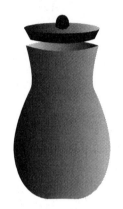

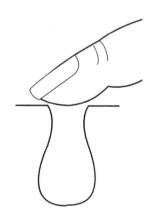

Tsubo

When we feel aches or pains, our natural response is to touch the painful area to find the exact source of pain. Simple pressure or rubbing these points often can ease the pain. The conceptualization of *tsubo* occurred over 3,000 to 10,000 years ago in the areas of China, northern India, Nepal, and Tibet in response to the discovery that certain painful points located on the body were common in all people. Since that time, *tsubo* became well-developed and systematized. It forms the foundation for massage, traditional Chinese medicine, and anma.

Tsubo is often translated as "acupoint" or "acupuncture point." In this book, I refer to these as *tsubo*. *Tsubo* are points on the body that can be used for to relieve pain or produce certain effects on the internal organs to relieve symptoms. Using *tsubo* and *keiraku* can be very effective with anma treatment.

The character for *tsubo* originated in China at least 3,000 years ago. It is a Chinese hieroglyph that literally translates as "jar." On the body, a *tsubo* is shaped something like a jar or deep pore.

One important concept of traditional Northeast Asian medicine is to imagine things in the universe that are invisible to the eye, such as air. Imagine the *tsubo* as small jars right beneath the skin which are filled with stagnant *ki*. Your fingertips are like lids, but they also have the power to go into the *tsubo* and rejuvenate the stagnating *ki*.

In treating *tsubo*, you apply pressure with your fingertips. Imagine opening the *tsubo* by first applying a light pressure. Next, imagine entering into the body applying a deep, firm pressure into the *tsubo*. Finally imagine closing the *tsubo* with last pressure. Opening the *tsubo* is very much like cutting into the body, and closure is very important so that the tsubo is not left exposed. An open *tsubo* is much like an open wound. Anma and shiatsu require that the full cycle be completed for effective therapy.

The concept of *tsubo* is one of the most important concepts for the effective use of anma during a treatment. The pressure application to the appropriate *tsubo* in anma and shiatsu ensures the release of the stagnating *ki*. Throughout this book, each treatment is based upon locating the proper *tsubo* and applying the appropriate pressure.

It is helpful to visualize a meridian as a hose with water running through it. The liquid (*toeki*) carries (*ki*) throughout the body. A *tsubo* is the point where stagnation commonly occurs on the meridian, just as kinks prevent water from flowing freely through a hose.

There are two categories of *tsubo*: *keiketsu* (*tsubo* on top of twelve meridians and two vessels), and *kiketsu* (*tsubo* not on the meridians, of which there are about 750 on each side of the body). The study of *tsubo*, however, is focused mainly on the *keiketsu*. There are about 361 *keiketsu tsubo* on each side of the body (see the table for the number of *tsubo* on each meridian). They can be thought of as a stagnation or counterpoint of the meridian.

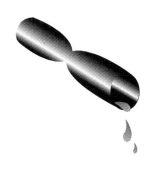

The precise location of *tsubo* is essential for treatment. Some *tsubo* are smaller than others, and if the practitioner is off by even one-sixteenth of an inch, effective treatment is not possible. *Tsubo* are generally located near the tip of a nerve or at a weak spot on the body, such as between the muscles and bones. *Tsubo* are normally located in slight depressions or indentations on the body. Through physical examination, these depressions can help you to locate the exact spot of the *tsubo*. The best way to learn the location of *tsubo* is to identify them on your own body. With this approach, you can feel the different sensations of pain and pressure at each point while learning the precise location of *tsubo* on the body.

Pain on a particular *tsubo* is often an indication of some irregularity in the physical or internal organs. Slightly different symptoms occur in each individual because each body is different. The response to the treatment to the *tsubo* varies as well.

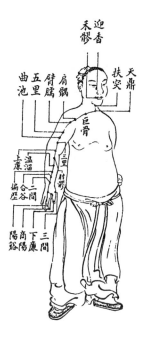

Tsubo, meridians, and all concepts of traditional Northeast Asian medicines require more intensive study to fully understand and perform. You must first diagnose conditions using pulse or abdominal diagnosis—an essential part of traditional Northeast Asian medical treatment. You must also have a deep understanding of Northeast Asian medical theory, meridians, and *tsubo*. Basic knowledge of Western anatomy, physiology, and pathology is helpful, but not necessary. In-depth study of meridians and *tsubo* in traditional Northeast Asian medicine can take a few years.

Out of the 361 points of *tsubo*, most acupuncturists and traditional Northeast Asian bodyworkers commonly use 130 to 200 for treatment. Other points are used for less common circumstances, but it's rare for a practitioner to use all *tsubo* points in one treatment. There are certain *tsubo* commonly used to treat an array of illnesses, while other points are used for such obscure conditions that therapists rarely use them.

Treatments using meridians and *tsubo* can enhance a practitioner's massage—but only after the hand manipulation techniques are well developed. Most people enjoy and benefit from a massage without the deeper understanding of the meridians and *tsubo*.

Listed below are the number of *tsubo* in each meridian:

Lung	11
Large Intestine	20
Stomach	45
Spleen	21
Heart	9
Small Intestine	19
Bladder	67
Kidney	27
Shin Po	9
San Sho	23
Gall Bladder	44
Liver	14
Nin Myaku	24
Toku Myaku	28

Meridians and *Tsubo* on the Face

The six *yang* meridians that pass through the face are the Large Intestine, Stomach, Small Intestine, Bladder, *San Sho*, and Gall Bladder Meridians. There are also two vessels, the Governing Vessel and the Conception Vessel, which run along the face.

Twelve of the *kei* meridians are divided into two categories with *Yin/Yang* Theory: six *yin* meridians and six *yang* meridians. They can also be divided into five categories with the Five Element Theory. These are fire, earth, metal, water, and wood.

Yin meridians correspond to the most vital organs of the body, Heart, Liver, Lung, Kidney, and Spleen (in terminology, the Asian "Spleen" closely corresponds to the Western "pancreas"). *Yang* meridians correspond to Large Intestines, Gall Bladder, Bladder, Stomach, and Small Intestines. The main function of *yang* meridians is to support the functioning of *yin* meridians of corresponding elements.

Only the *yang* meridians reach above the neck, and all six *yang* meridians meet at the face. Three *yang* meridians of the arm start at the fingertips and end at the face. The other three *yang* meridians, the leg meridians, start around the eye and run across the body to end at the toes. As I explained earlier, the face is the place of transition for *yang* meridians, and it is essential for human health that the *ki* flow from the end of one meridian to the beginning of the other is kept in smooth transition.

For example, the Large Intestine Meridian finishes at the side of the nose but connects to the Stomach Meridian just beneath the center of the lower eyelid. In order to reach the Stomach Meridian, the *ki* must flow upward along the side of the nose to the medial corner of the eye, and then downward and out along the lower eyelid to reach the starting point of the Stomach Meridian. This area between the two meridians is not itself a meridian but rather a connecting area between the two which contributes to the efficiency of *ki* flow between the two meridians.

The next three pages show three different views of the meridians on the face and the head. It is difficult to describe in words or pictures since the head is three-dimensional. It can be rather complicated, so the pages that follow describe each meridian, one by one, and the corresponding *tsubo*.

For further study of the meridian system and *tsubo*, traditional meridian dolls are very helpful study aids.

See the back of this book for details.

Keiraku (Meridians) on the Face
Lateral view

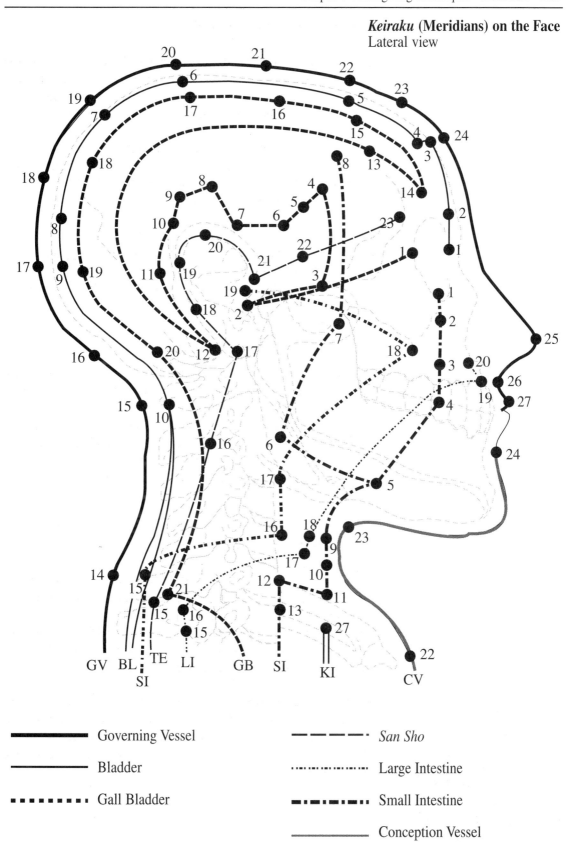

——— Governing Vessel	– – – – – *San Sho*
——— Bladder	·············· Large Intestine
■■■■■■ Gall Bladder	–·–·–·–· Small Intestine
	~~ Conception Vessel

Keiraku (Meridians) on the Face
Anterior view

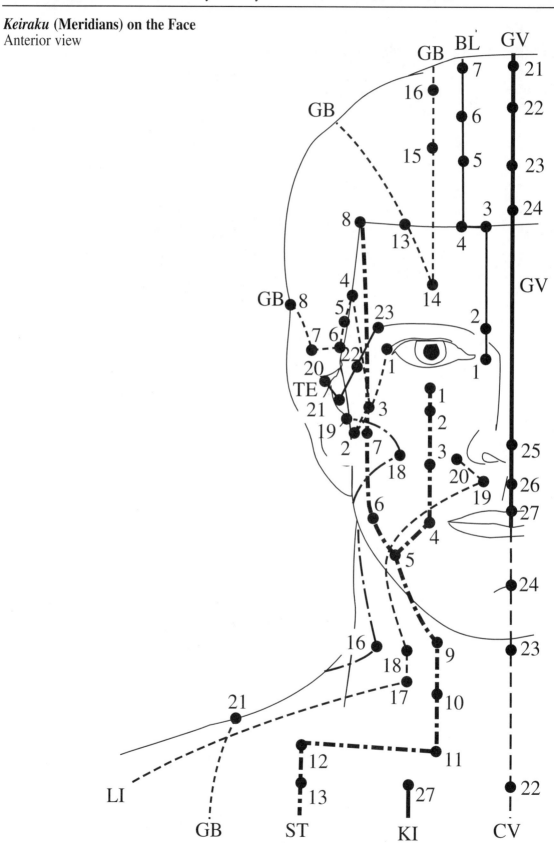

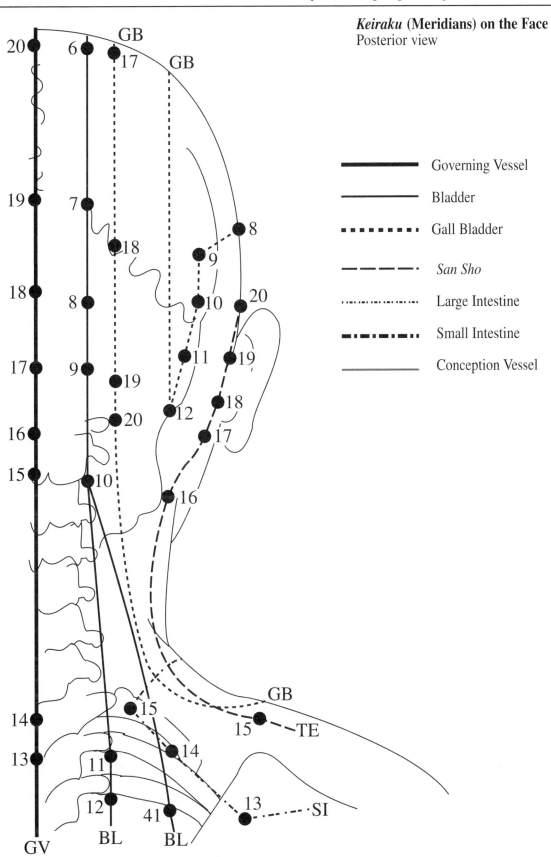

***Keiraku* (Meridians) on the Face**
Posterior view

Legend:
- Governing Vessel
- Bladder
- Gall Bladder
- *San Sho*
- Large Intestine
- Small Intestine
- Conception Vessel

Dai Cho Kei—Large Intestine Meridian

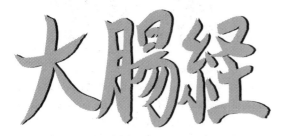

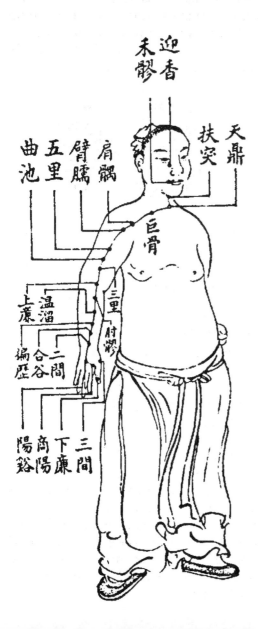

The Function of the Large Intestine Meridian

The main function of the Large Intestine Meridian is to support the functioning of the large intestine. The Large Intestine is responsible for separating liquid and solid waste and then eliminating the final solid waste. It also is responsible for the waste from the internal body such as in the blood and the circulatory system.

In traditional Japanese medical theory, Lung refers to the entire system that works to handle the intake and exhaust of air. The Lungs and Large Intestine are closely related (*yin* and *yang* in the metal element), supporting and affecting one another. The throat and nasal passages are closely connected to the Lungs and Large Intestines.

The Lung is also in charge of "defensive *ki*," which is similar to the Western concept of an "immune system": both are the primary defenses against illness that enters the body. If the Lung detects any sign of illness, it conveys this to the Large Intestine, which causes diarrhea or constipation.

Pathways of the Large Intestine Meridian

The Large Intestine Meridian starts at the radial side of the base of the index fingernail (*sho yo*, Large Intestine-1) and travels up the radial side of the finger to the radial side of the second metacarpal. It continues to the meeting of the first and second metacarpals (*go koku*, Large Intestine-4), across the radial back of the hand and forearm, and up the triceps to the center of the deltoid. Next, it moves up the shoulder and travels along the highest point of the suprascapular region, across the front of the neck to the side of the mouth and finally finishes at the base and side of the nose (*gei ko*, Large Intestine-20).

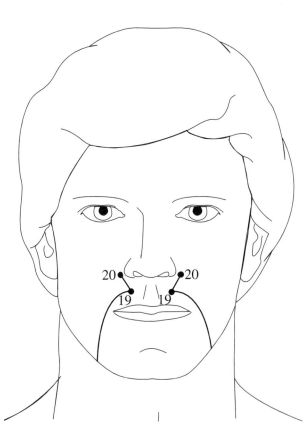

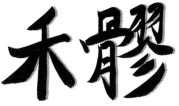

ka ryo (Large Intestine-19)

Ka means "grain" and *ryo* means "bone" or "indentation of bone." Together they mean "grainy indentation of bone." *Ka ryo* is located midway between the nostril and upper lip, directly inferior to the nostril. You will feel the indentation on the gum directly superior to the front teeth. *Ka ryo* is used in Japanese facial massage to improve the appearance of the region between the nostril and the upper lip. This point is also used for improving the air flow within the nose, the condition of clogged nasal passages, and nosebleeding.

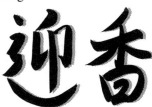

gei ko (Large Intestine-20)

Gei means "welcome" and *ko* means "fragrant." Together they mean "welcoming fragrance." Among the Five Elements Theory of five smells (rancid, burned, fragrant, fishy, and putrid,) *ko* is the third smell, "fragrant," which corresponds to Earth Elements. *Gei ko* is the last point of the Large Intestine Meridian and the meeting point of stomach and large intestine meridians. *Gei ko* also translates to "welcoming the stomach meridians or earth element meridians (stomach and spleen)." This *tsubo* is found slightly (half a thumb-width) lateral to the nare.

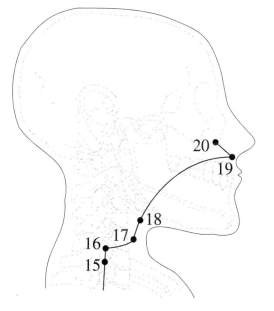

Light stimulation to *gei ko* is often used in Japanese facial massage to improve appearance and help prevent wrinkles around the nostril region. *Gei ko* is used to help relieve clogged nasal passages, loss of the sense of smell, runny nose, allergic rhinitis, and many other nose-related problems. Both *ka ryo* and *gei ko* are used to prevent wrinkles around the crease between the nose and the corner of the lips (nasolabial crease).

Japanese Facial-Massage Techniques—Example #26

Pressure to *Tsubo* on the Large Intestine Meridian

Japanese name of this technique

指頭圧迫法

shi to ap paku ho

0°

Center Position

The purpose of this technique

Improve appearance around the sides of the mouth and nose

Area of application

Crease along the outer sides of the mouth to the side of the nose (nasolabial groove)

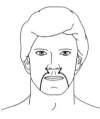

Description

Dai cho kei (Large Intestine Meridian) begins at the index finger and runs across and behind the arm to the top of the shoulder. From there it runs up to the crease along the outer edge of the mouth, and ends just to the side of the nostril. Two *tsubo* of the Large Intestine Meridian are found in the face, and *gei ko* (Large Intestine-20) is an especially important *tsubo* to remember. Stimulating these *tsubo* helps improve the appearance around the area from the sides of the nose to the mouth.

No Lubrication

All examples in this chapter are demonstrated on the right side of the face. You should always work both sides of the face evenly, one after another. The hand that is not being used to massage the face should provide light support to stabilize the head.

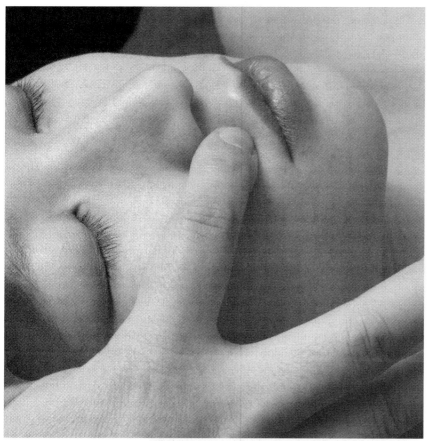

1 Lightly rest the heel of your right hand against the right side of the client's face, around the area in front of the ear. Apply pressure to the *ka ryo* (Large Intestine-19) with the tip of your index finger. *Ka ryo* is found at the midpoint between the nostril and the upper lip, directly inferior to the nostril. Hold gentle pressure while the client is exhaling for two to five seconds, then release. Repeat several times or as many times as desired.

2 Move the tip of the index finger and apply pressure to *gei ko* (Large Intestine-20). *Gei ko* is found slightly (a half thumb-width) lateral to the nare. Hold gentle pressure while the client is exhaling for two to five seconds, then release. Repeat several times or as many times as desired.

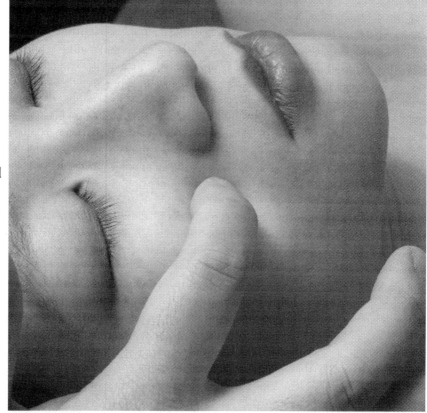

Japanese Facial-Massage Techniques—Example #27

Stroking the Large Intestine Meridian

Japanese name of this technique

二指軽擦法

ni shi kei satsu ho

The purpose of this technique

Improve the appearance around the side areas of the mouth and nose

Area of application

Crease along the outer sides of the mouth to the side of the nose (nasolabial groove)

Description

The crease that runs along either side of the mouth is a common place to develop wrinkles. As a person ages, these wrinkles tend to deepen. In this area, massaging with upward strokes—working from the jaw line toward the nose—helps prevent wrinkles as well as restore the natural elasticity of the skin.

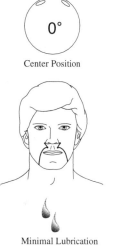

0°

Center Position

Minimal Lubrication

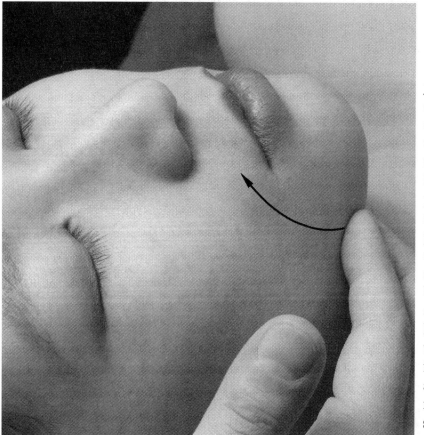

1 Lightly place the heel of your hand just in front of the client's ear. Follow the crease that runs along the side of the mouth to find the point where it meets the jaw. Place your index finger at the edge of the jaw. Lightly place the middle finger over the index finger so they slightly overlap. Use a slow, light stroke along the Large Intestine Meridian up toward the nose, following the crease along the outside of the mouth. **Do not pull the skin with the stroke.**

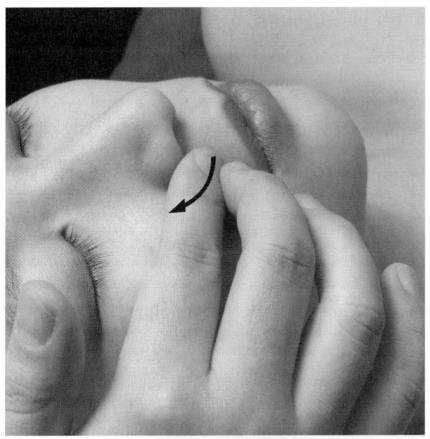

2 Continue with a slightly curved stroke around the side of the lips toward *ka ryo* (Large Intestine-19), which is directly below the nostril, midway between the nostril and the upper lip. Once you reach *ka ryo*, change the direction of the stroke toward *gei ko*.

3 Continue stroking until you reach *gei ko* (Large Intestine-20). *Gei ko* is found slightly (half a thumb-width) lateral to the nare. After reaching *gei ko*, return to Step 1 and repeat the sequence once or twice.

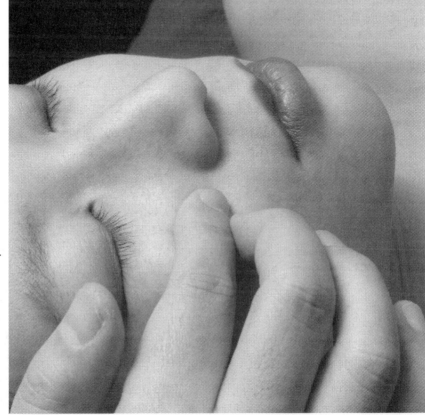

I Kei—Stomach Meridian

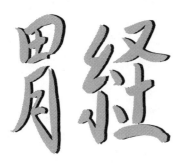

The Function of the Stomach Meridian

The main function of the Stomach Meridian is to support the functioning of the Stomach. The primary function of the Stomach is to receive and examine food (and if food is spoiled or toxic, to eject it), and then to break it down.

According to traditional Japanese medical theory, the Stomach extracts *sei ki* (approximate translation: "nutrition") from the food, and sends it to the Spleen. The remaining matter is sent to the Small Intestines.

The Stomach is closely related to the Spleen (the Northeast Asian term "Spleen" is similar to the Western term "pancreas"), and the two affect one another. The Spleen is in charge of distributing *sei ki*.

Pathway of the Stomach Meridian

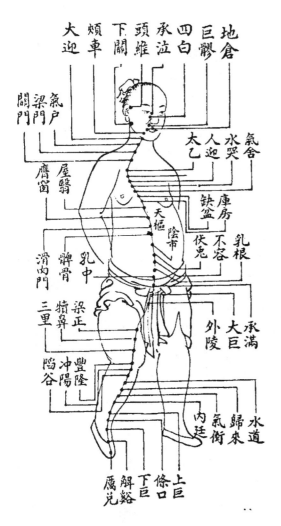

The Stomach Meridian begins at the bottom of the middle of the eye and follows straight down the cheekbone to the outside corner of the lips before angling to the middle of the cheekbone where it splits (Stomach-5). One fork follows the jawbone, runs up to the front of the ear, and continues up to the top corner of the forehead where it ends (Stomach-8). The other fork moves down from the jawbone and along the front of the throat to the top of the clavicle. From there, it moves laterally along the top to the middle of the clavicle and down the chest and abdomen between the Liver and Kidney Meridians.

At the base of the trunk, it runs laterally to the front of the leg and then down. It runs just lateral to the kneecap and just on the lateral side of the front of the tibia. Midway down, it juts to the lateral temporarily before continuing back down on the front of the leg and ankle. It finishes by running between the second and third metatarsal to the lateral corner of the second toenail, where it ends.

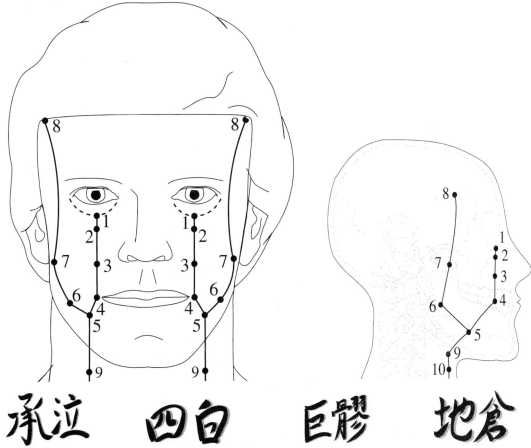

承泣
sho kyu
(Stomach-1)
Means "containing tears." This *tsubo* is often used to improve appearance of the eyes and to help prevent wrinkles around the eyes.

四白
shi haku
(Stomach-2)
Means "corner of hollow between eyes." Light stimulation of this *tsubo* improves the appearance of tissue just beneath the lower eyelid.

巨髎
ko ryo
(Stomach-3)
Means "large depression." Light stimulation of this *tsubo* improves the appearance on the cheek beside the nose.

地倉
chi so
(Stomach-4)
Means "stone house of the earth." Light stimulation of this *tsubo* improves appearance at corner of lips.

大迎
dai gei
(Stomach-5)
Means "great welcome." This *tsubo* is often used to improve appearance of the skin to the side of the chin along the jawline.

頰車
kyo sha
(Stomach-6)
Means "wheels of the chin or cheek." This *tsubo* is often used to improve appearance of the skin along the jawline between ear and chin.

下関
ge kan
(Stomach-7)
Means "lower of separated parts." This *tsubo* is often used to reduce inflammation of the TMJ.

頭維
zu i
(Stomach-8)
Means "support the head." This *tsubo* is often used to help prevent hair loss and to help relieve headaches and migraines.

Japanese Facial-Massage Techniques—Example #28

Pressure to *Tsubo* on the Stomach Meridian

Japanese name for this technique

0°

Center Position

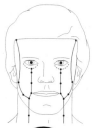

No Lubrication

指頭圧迫法

shi to ap paku ho

The purpose of this technique

Improve the appearance under the eyes, over the cheek, and along the jaw

Area of application

Tsubo on the *i kei* (Stomach Meridian)

Description

The *tsubo* on the Stomach Meridian has close associations with the cheek region beneath the eye and along edge of jaw. Light stimulation of these *tsubo* can improve appearance and prevent wrinkles at the top of cheekbones. Application of pressure to *sho kyu* (Stomach-1) has been omitted in this book, due to its closeness to the eye.

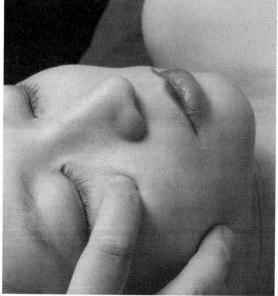

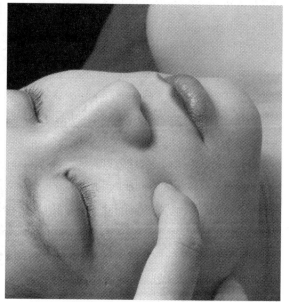

1 Lightly place the tips of the thumb and middle finger on the side of the client's face to stabilize the hand. Apply pressure with the index finger to *shi haku* (Stomach-2). This *tsubo* is found one thumb-width directly inferior to the pupil at the upper edge of the cheekbone (infraorbital region).

2 Keep the tips of the thumb and middle fingers in the same position. Apply pressure with the index finger to *ko ryo* (Stomach-3). *Ko ryo* is found directly below the pupil, a half thumb-width lateral to the *gei ko* (Large Intestine-20) and level with the bottom of the nose.

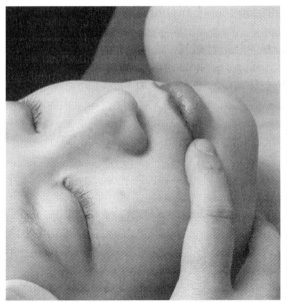

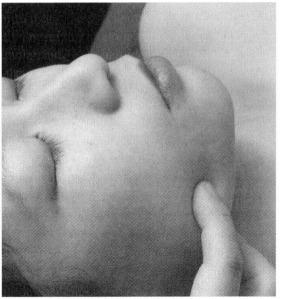

3 Keep the tips of the thumb and middle fingers in the same position. Apply gentle pressure with the index finger to *chi so* (Stomach-4). This *tsubo* is found slightly lateral to the edge of the lips when they are closed naturally. Hold pressure while the client is exhaling for two to five seconds, then release.

4 Apply pressure with the index finger to *dai gei* (Stomach-5). This *tsubo* is found in the depression on the edge of the jawbone (mandible) and level with the crease of the chin, where you can feel the pulse. Adjust the position of your thumb and middle fingers as needed to keep the hand stabilized.

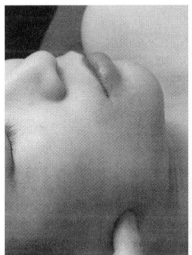

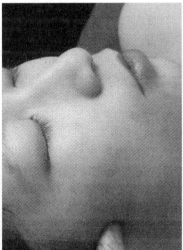

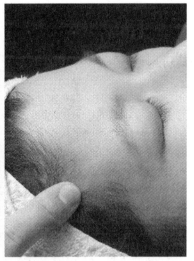

5 Move the hand and lightly place it onto the neck. Apply pressure with the index finger to *kyo sha* (Stomach-6). This *tsubo* is on the edge of the jawbone about one thumb-width below the earlobe, in the depression of the masseter muscle.

6 Move the hand over the ear. Apply pressure with the index finger to *ge kan* (Stomach-7). This *tsubo* is found just inferior to the cheekbone, slightly toward the eye from the molar, and disappears when the mouth opens.

7 Move the hand over the head. Apply pressure with the index finger to *zu i* (Stomach-8). This *tsubo* is found in the slight depression at the corner of the natural hairline of the forehead.

Japanese Facial-Massage Techniques—Example #29

Stroking the Stomach Meridian

Center Position

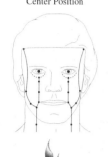

Minimal Lubrication

Japanese name for this technique

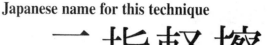

ni shi kei satsu ho

The purpose of this technique

Improve appearance around the cheek region

Area of application

Over the cheek, along the jaw, and up to the forehead

Description

This technique lightly strokes along the Stomach Meridian.

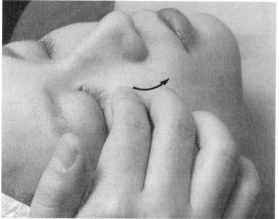

1 Place slightly overlapping index and middle fingers at *shi haku* (Stomach-2), found one thumb-width directly inferior the pupil at the upper edge of the cheekbone (infraorbital region). Lightly stroke down the cheek toward *ko ryo* (Stomach-3), found directly below the pupil, a half thumb-width lateral from the *gei ko* (Large Intestine-20) and is level with the bottom of the nose.

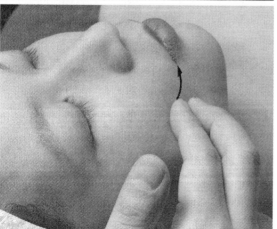

2 Stroke toward *chi so* (Stomach-4), found slightly outside the edge of the lips when they are closed naturally.

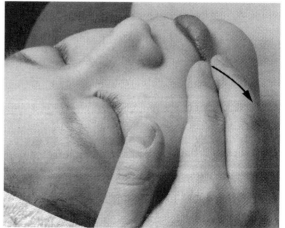

3 From *chi so* (Stomach-4), stroke outward to *dai gei* (Stomach-5), which is found in the depression on the edge of the jawbone and is level with the crease of the chin.

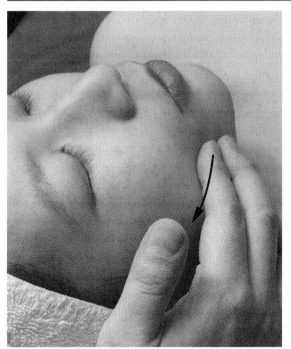

4 Continue stroking from *dai gei* (Stomach-5), toward *kyo sha* (Stomach-6), located on the edge of the jawbone about one thumb-width below the earlobe in the depression of the masseter muscle.

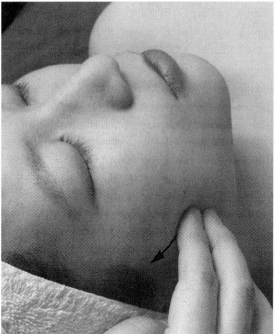

5 Stroke upward from *kyo sha* (Stomach-6) toward *ge kan* (Stomach-7), which is found just under the cheekbone, slightly toward the eye from the molar.

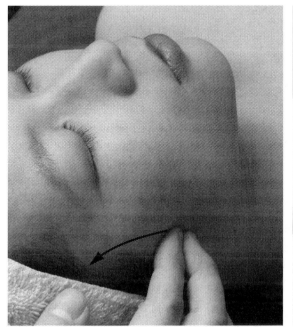

6 Continue stroking from *ge kan* (Stomach-7), moving upward over the cheek to *zu i* (Stomach-8), found in the slight depression at the corner of the natural hairline of the forehead.

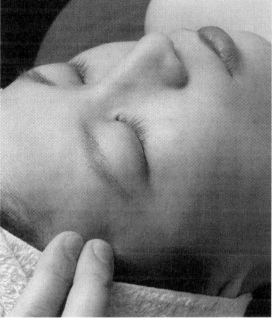

7 Stop stroking when you reach *zu i* (Stomach-8). Repeat several times, as desired, by returning to the starting position.

Sho Cho Kei—Small Intestine Meridian

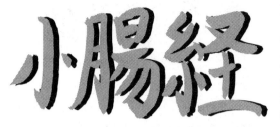

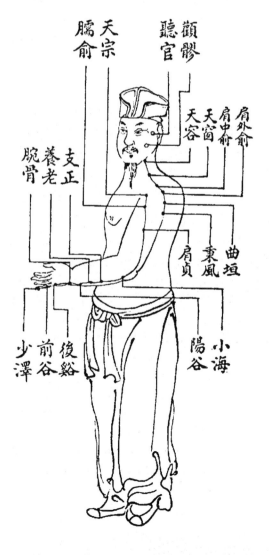

Function of the Small Intestine Meridian

The main function of the Small Intestine Meridian is to support the Small Intestine. The primary function of the Small Intestine is to separate *sei ki* (which is close to the Western concept of nutrition) and *zan sa* (leftover waste). Once separated, the Small Intestine sends *sei ki* to the Spleen and *zan sa* to the Large Intestine.

The Small Intestine has a close relation to the heart: one of its primary functions is to support the functioning of the Heart. The Heart is the most important organ, and the Small Intestine is the primary energetic source for the heart. In traditional Japanese theory, the Small Intestine is called the origin of *ki*, the very center of the *hara* (the abdomen).

If the Small Intestine does not function properly, it may cause diarrhea and blood in the stool or urine; these symptoms can also be caused by excessive heat in the Heart.

Pathway of the Small Intestine Meridian

The Small Intestine Meridian begins at the posterior side of the the tip of the fifth finger. It travels up the finger to the hand and stays between the fourth and the fifth metacarpals to the wrist. The Small Intestine Meridian continues along the posteriomedial aspect of the lower and upper arms, passes through the back of the shoulder and zigzags across the shoulder blade. It then travels up the back of the suprascapula to the base of the neck, across the sternocleidomastoid, and up to the corner of the cheekbone. It finishes on the tab (tragus) of the ear (*cho kyu*, Small Intestine-19).

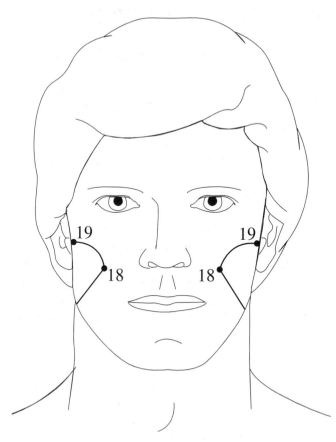

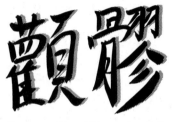

kan ryo (Small Intestine-18)
Kan means "cheekbone" and *ryo* means "indentation on the bone." This *tsubo* is found in the depression just below the cheekbone (zygomatic bone), level with the bottom of the nose. *Kan ryo* means "indentation just under cheekbone." This is one of the most important *tsubo* in the treatment of facial beauty: it helps sustain the firmness of the entire musculature within the cheek and prevent wrinkles on the region from the bottom of the eye to the side of the mouth. Light stimulation to this *tsubo* can improve the appearance of the entire cheek.

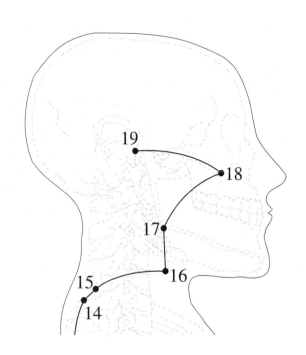

cho kyu (Small Intestine-19)
Cho means "listen" and *kyu* means "palace." Together they mean "palace of listening." This *tsubo* is found in the depression just in front of the tragus (the tab of the ear), between *cho e* (Gall Bladder-2) and *ji mon* (*San Sho*-21). *Cho kyu* is used to treat all kinds of ear-related problems. It is one of the most effective points in the treatment of tinnitus and difficulty in hearing, and it is also used to relieve headaches and dizziness.

Pressure to *Tsubo* on the Small Intestine Meridian

Japanese name for this technique

指頭圧迫法

shi to ap paku ho

0°

Center Position

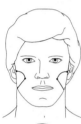

No Lubrication

The purpose of this technique

Improve the appearance of the tissue on the side of the cheek, in front of the ear, as well as muscular firmness in the cheeks

Area of application

Side of the cheek, in front of the ear over the Small Intestine Meridian

Description

Sho cho kei (Small Intestine Meridian) is closely related to the condition of the digestive system, along with *i kei* (Stomach Meridian) and *dai cho kei* (Large Intestine Meridian). *Sho cho kei* is connected to the Small Intestines and the Heart, both of which are fire elements. It contributes to the primary *ki*, the energy that supports bodily functions.

The conditions of the Small Intestine and Heart Meridians are closely related with the condition of the facial skin. Proper functioning of these meridians results in a very rich, warm facial tone. Irregularities of these meridians or of the Kidney Meridian often result in a pale, whitish tone or dark complexion. For severe instances of these cases, I recommend treatment of these meridians throughout the body, not just on the face. Signs of irregularity in the *sho cho kei* often appear in the cheek: if it is excessive (*jitsu*), cheek tissue becomes very tight, stiff, and dry; if it is depleted (*kyo*), cheek tissue becomes loose and watery.

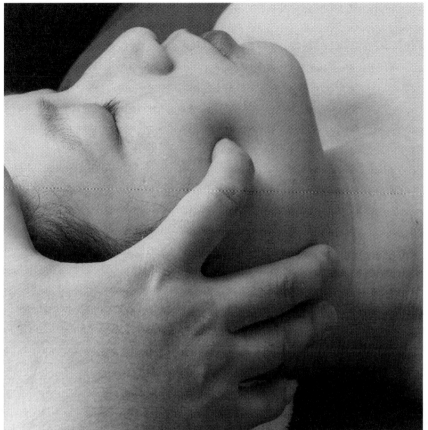

1 Lightly place your hand over the ear so that the index and ring fingers and the thumb stabilize the hand. Apply pressure to *kan ryo* (Small Intestine-18) with the tip of the index finger. *Kan ryo* is found in the depression just below the cheekbone (zygomatic bone), level with the bottom of the nose.

2 Move your hand over the client's head, stabilizing it again with the index and ring fingers and the thumb. Apply pressure to *cho kyu* (Small Intestine-19) with the tip of the index finger. *Cho kyu* is found in the depression just in front of the ear tab, between *cho e* (Gall Bladder-2) and *ji mon* (*San Sho*-21).

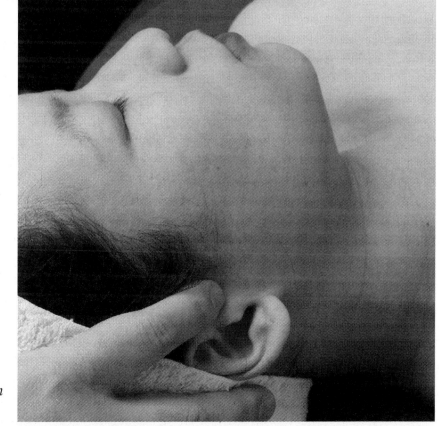

Japanese Facial-Massage Techniques—Example #31

Stroking the Small Intestine Meridian

Japanese name for this technique

二指軽擦法

ni shi kei satsu ho

0°

Center Position

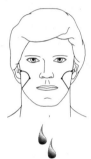

Minimal Lubrication

The purpose of this technique

Improve the appearance of the regions on the side of the cheek in front of the ear, as well as muscle firmness in the cheeks

Area of application

Side of the cheek, in front of the ear over the Small Intestine Meridian

Description

Stroking the Small Intestine Meridian is an excellent way to improve the facial appearance of regions on the hollows of the cheeks. You can use slightly heavier pressure during the upstroke, but do not pull the skin.

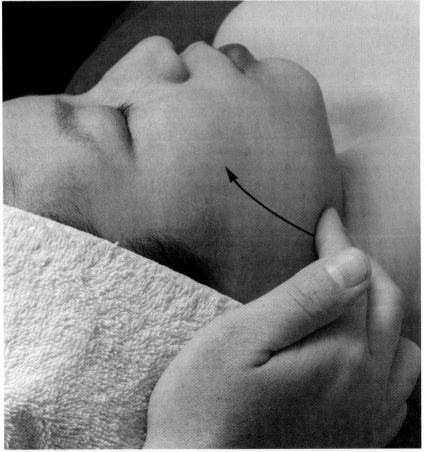

1 Lightly place the heel of your hand just behind the client's eye to stabilize the hand. Place the index finger on the back edge of the jawbone, two to three thumb-widths under the ear. Lightly place the middle finger over the index finger so they slightly overlap. Slowly stroke along the Small Intestine Meridian toward the center of the cheek.

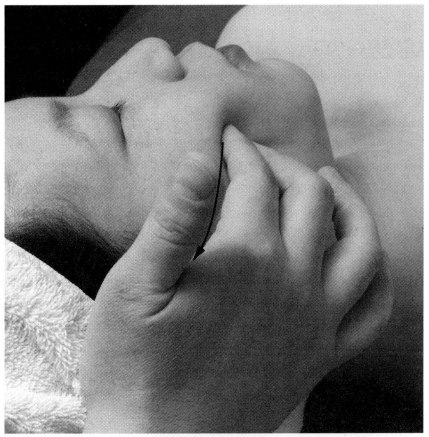

2 Continue stroking until you reach the *kan ryo* (Small Intestine-18). This *tsubo* is found in the depression just below the cheekbone, directly inferior to the lateral corner of the eye. Once you have reached *kan ryo*, change the direction of the stroke toward the ear tab, gently following the contour of the cheek. Again, use very light press in your stroke.

3 Continue stroking until you reach the *cho kyu* (Small Intestine-19). This *tsubo* is found in the depression just anterior to the ear tab, in between *cho e* (Gall Bladder-2) and *ji mon* (San Sho-21). Repeat two to three times by returning to your starting position.

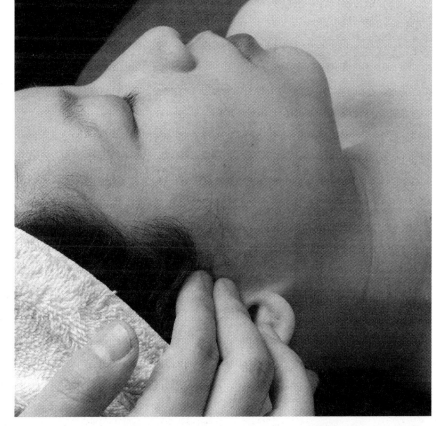

Bo Ko Kei—Bladder Meridian

膀胱経

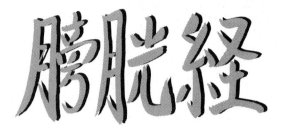

Function of the Bladder Meridian

The main function of the Bladder Meridian is to support the bladder. The Small Intestine receives a nutritionally rich liquid from the Stomach, and determines how much nutrition must be extracted and circulated throughout the body. What is not needed is eliminated as sweat or sent to the Bladder to be expelled as urine. The Bladder receives liquid waste from the Small Intestine and other internal organs, which it holds and releases back into the body as needed. When the Bladder reaches full capacity, it attempts to empty itself through the urinary tract.

The Kidneys are closely related to the Bladder, which are *yin* and *yang* in the Water Element. The Kidneys (which produce one of the most important types of *ki*) function optimally when the Bladder is healthy; when the Bladder is out of balance, the Kidneys are not able to function properly.

Pathway of the Bladder Meridian

The Bladder Meridian begins at the inner corner of the eye (Bladder-1). It travels up to the inner corners of the eyebrows (Bladder-2), up the forehead, and over and behind the head. At the base of the skull (*ten chu*, Bladder-10) it splits, with one side running lateral to the spine and the other running lateral to the erector muscles; both travel down to the buttocks. The Inner Bladder Meridian travels down the base of the buttocks and down the back of the leg. The Outer Bladder Meridian runs down the back of the gluteus maximus and down the back of the leg lateral to the Inner Bladder Meridian. The two join just above the knee and continue down the back of the calf, lateral to the Achilles tendon and under the ankle bone, and along the lateral and dorsal sides of the foot. This is the longest meridian in the body.

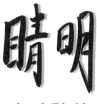

sei mei (Bladder-1)

Sei means "iris" or "pupil" and *mei* mean "brightness." This *tsubo* is located in the corner of the eye, just on the bridge of the nose. This is used to beautify, refresh, and brighten the eyes.

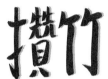

san chiku (Bladder-2)

San means "together" and *chiku* means "bamboo" (bamboo often indicates hair of eyebrow). *San chiku* is located in depression of medial edge of eyebrow. Light stimulation of this point helps to prevent and reduce wrinkles between eyebrows. This *tsubo* also relieves headaches and high blood pressure.

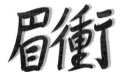

bi sho (Bladder-3)

Bi means "eyebrow" and *sho* means "balancing." *Bi sho* is located in depression superior to *san chiku* on the hairline. It is used to prevent hair loss, relieve headaches, and balance emotions.

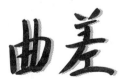

kyoku sa (Bladder-4)

Kyoku means "bend" and *sa* means "differential." *Kyoku sa* is found in the depression one thumb-width lateral from *bi sho*, on the hairline. It is used to prevent hair loss and relieve headaches.

Japanese Facial-Massage Techniques—Example #32

Pressure to *Tsubo* on the Bladder Meridian

Japanese name for this technique

指頭圧迫法

shi to ap paku ho

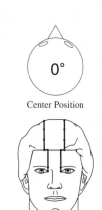

0°

Center Position

No Lubrication

The purpose of this technique

Improve appearance in the region between the eyebrows to the center of the forehead

Area of application

Medial corner of the eye and the center of the forehead region along the Bladder Meridian

Description

Bo ko kei (Bladder Meridian) and *jin kei* (Kidney Meridian) belong to the water elements and are closely related to the condition of the body fluids and liquids.

Treatment of the Bladder Meridian is good for improving the appearance between the eyes and the middle of the forehead, but it also helps balance the level of moisture in facial skin. Light stimulation to these points and stroking of Bladder Meridian helps remoisturize dry skin with body fluids or helps drain excess fluids from overmoist skin. For severe conditions, combine facial massage with an entire body treatment such as anma, shiatsu, or acupuncture.

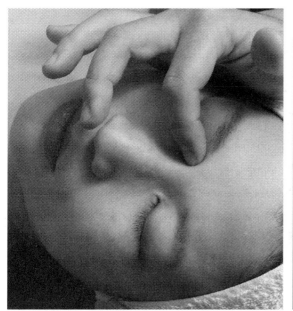

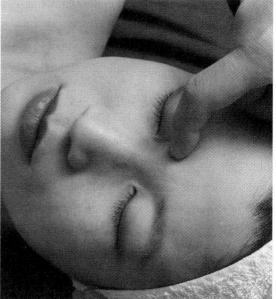

1 Lightly place the heel of your hand in front of the client's ear to stabilize the hand. Apply gentle pressure to the *sei mei* (Bladder-1) with the index finger. *Sei mei* is found in the depression on the medial corner of the eye on the side of the bridge of the nose.

2 Move the hand toward the top of the head to stabilize it. Apply gentle pressure to the *san chiku* (Bladder-2) with the index finger for three to five seconds, then release. *San chiku* is found in the depression on the medial end of the eyebrow.

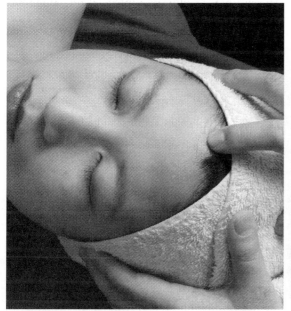

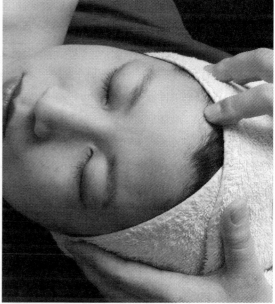

3 Move the hand more toward the center of the top of the head. Apply pressure to the *bi sho* (Bladder-3) with the index finger. *Bi sho* is found in the depression superior to *san chiku* on the hairline.

4 Apply pressure to the *kyoku sa* (Bladder-4) with the index finger. *Kyoku sa* is found in the depression outside, one thumb-width from *bi sho*. Hold gentle pressure while the client is exhaling for two to five seconds, then release. Repeat several times or as often as desired.

Japanese Facial-Massage Techniques—Example #33

Stroking the Bladder Meridian

Japanese name for this technique

二指軽擦法

ni shi kei satsu ho

0°

Center Position

The purpose of this technique

Improve the appearance in the region between the eyebrows to the center of the forehead

Area of application

Medial corner of the eye and the center of the forehead region along the Bladder Meridian

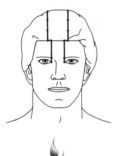

Minimal Lubrication

Description

When you are stroking the forehead, you can apply slightly heavier pressure, since the bone is so close to the surface of the skin. When you are stroking right next to the eye, use caution not to touch the eyeball or spread lubricant onto the eye tissue. Use enough lubrication to prevent pulling the client's skin.

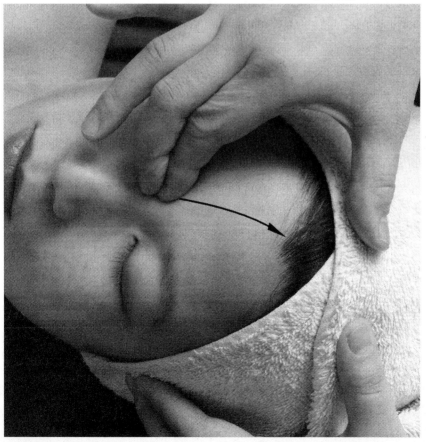

1 Place your thumb in the depression just above the client's forehead. Apply pressure to *sei mei* (Bladder-1) with the index finger. This *tsubo* is found in the depression on the medial corner of the eye on the side of the bridge of the nose. Stroke toward *san chiku* (Bladder-2) at the inner edge of the eyebrow and continue stroking upward on the forehead toward *bi sho* (Bladder-3).

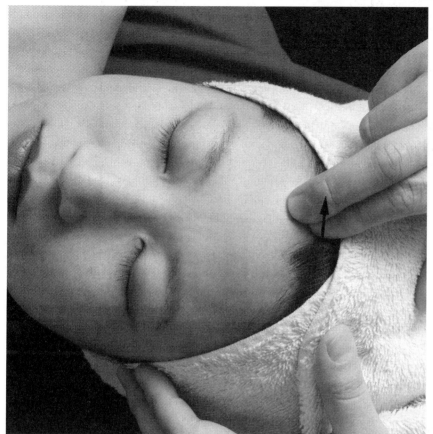

2 You can slightly readjust the position of the thumb as necessary to bring the stroke upward. Stroke from *bi sho* (Bladder-3) to *kyoku sa* (Bladder-4) with the index finger. This stroke is one thumb-width lateral from the center line along the hairline. Minimize the amount of lubricant that goes into the hair.

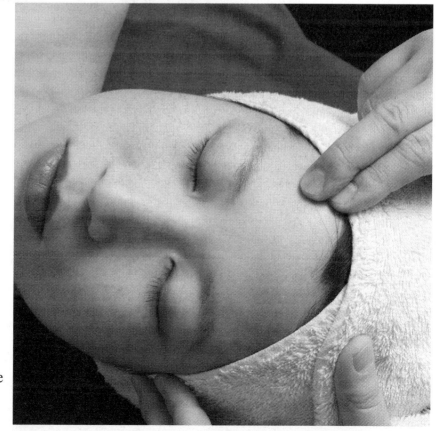

3 End the stroke at *kyoku sa* (Bladder-4). Repeat two to three times by returning to the starting position.

San Sho Kei—San Sho Meridian

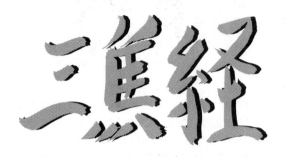

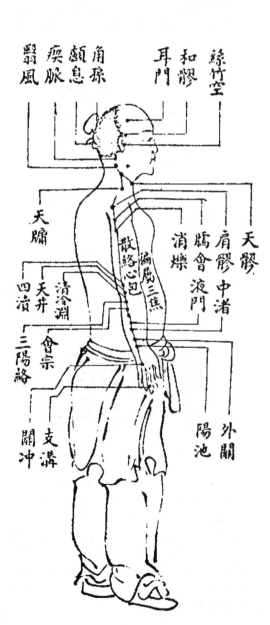

Function of the *San Sho* Meridian

San means "three" and *sho* means "roasting" or "heating." The typical translation is "triple burner" or "triple heater" (to avoid confusion among the many translations for this word, we will refer to this simply as *San Sho*). Western medical theory does not have an organ which corresponds to the *San Sho* Meridian. It is responsible for the distribution of circulatory fluids (traditionally "blood," "liquid," and "fluid"), and aids the digestive system. In addition to this, the *San Sho* Meridian clears circulatory passages, and the body can remain pure through proper circulatory functions. The waste matter picked up by the *San Sho* Meridian is sent to the Large Intestine and Bladder for elimination.

The *san sho* is a multifunctional organ; it distributes its work among three "burners." The Upper Burner is related to the Heart and Lungs; the Middle Burner is related to the Spleen and Stomach; and the Lower Burner is related to the Liver, Small intestine, Large Intestine, Kidneys, and Bladder. The *San Sho* Meridian is also closely related to the *shin po* (similar to "pericardium") and the Heart.

Pathway of the *San Sho* Meridian

The *San Sho* Meridian begins at the tip of the fourth finger and travels up the back of the finger and between the fourth and fifth metacarpals on the back of the hand. It then travels past the wrist on the posterior side of the forearm and upper arm, over the back and side of the shoulder, and up the back of the suprascapula to the base of the neck. From here, it travels up the side of the neck to the earlobe and around behind the ear, attaching to the top of the head, and finishes at the outer edge of the eyebrow.

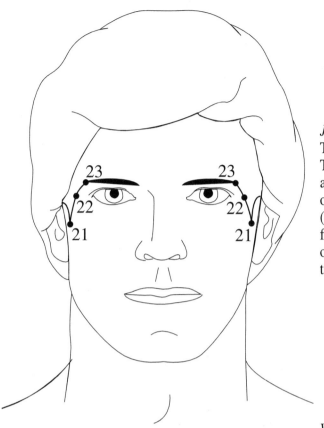

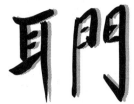

ji mon (*San Sho*-21)
Ji means "ear" and *mon* means "gate." Together they mean "gate of the ear." This *tsubo* is found in the depression just anterior to the upper attachment of the ear, one thumb-width superior the *cho kyu* (Small Intestine-19). It is used to improve facial appearance in the region in front of the ears and to relieve headaches and tinnitus.

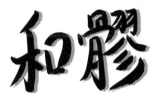

wa ryo (*San Sho*-22)
Wa means "harmony" and *ryo* means "indentation of bone." This *tsubo* is located in the depression on the temple, near the hairline where you can feel the pulse of the temporal artery. This *tsubo* harmonizes *ki* over the temporal region and helps to relieve tinnitus and headaches.

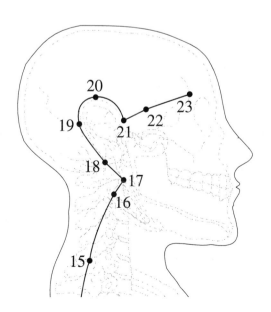

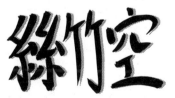

shi chiku ku (*San Sho*-23)
Shi means "silk," *chiku* means "bamboo" (this commonly indicates hair of eyebrow), and *ku* means "sky" or "empty." Together these mean "empty spot of eyebrow." This *tsubo* is found in the depression on the lateral edge of the eyebrow. *Shi chiku ku* harmonizes *ki* over the temporal region and helps to relieve headaches and treat psychosis.

Japanese Facial-Massage Techniques—Example #34

Pressure to *Tsubo* on the *San Sho* Meridian

Japanese name for this technique

0°

Center Position

指頭圧迫法

shi to ap paku ho

The purpose of this technique

Promote proper *ki* flow on the *San Sho* Meridian

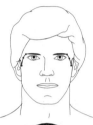

Area of application

Over the temple region along the *San Sho* Meridian

Description

These points (and the points behind the ear) on the *San Sho* Meridian are known to help with headaches and tinnitus (ringing in the ear). Stimulation of these *tsubo* is also used to help balance *ki* of the temporal region, which brings body and mind into harmony. Be sensitive when applying pressure here: too much pressure can cause headaches.

No Lubrication

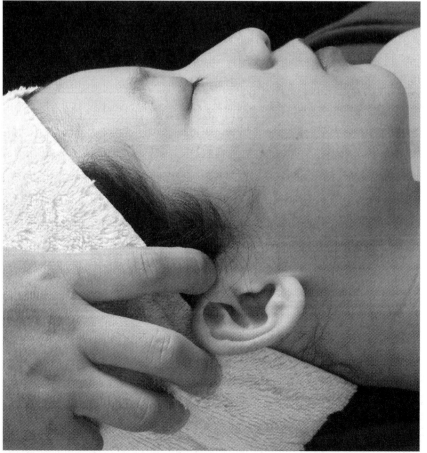

1 Lightly place your thumb, index, and middle fingers over the side of the client's head to stabilize the hand. Apply pressure to the *ji mon* (*San Sho*-21) with the index finger. *Ji mon* is found in the depression anterior to the upper attachment of the ear, one thumb-width superior to the *cho kyu* (Small Intestine-19).

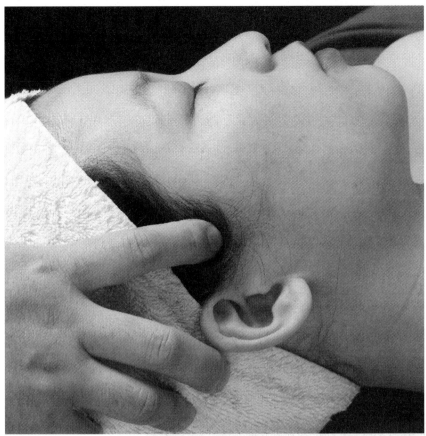

2 Adjust your hand as needed to keep it stabilized. Apply pressure to the *wa ryo* (*San Sho*-22) with the index finger. This *tsubo* is located in the depression on the temple, near the hairline where you can feel the pulse of the temporal artery. Hold gentle pressure while the client is exhaling for two to five seconds, then release. Repeat \several times or as many times as desired.

3 Apply pressure to the *shi chiku ku* (*San Sho*-23) with the index finger. *Shi chiku ku* is found in the depression on the lateral edge of the eyebrow. Hold gentle pressure while the client is exhaling for two to five seconds, then release. Repeat several times or as many times as desired.

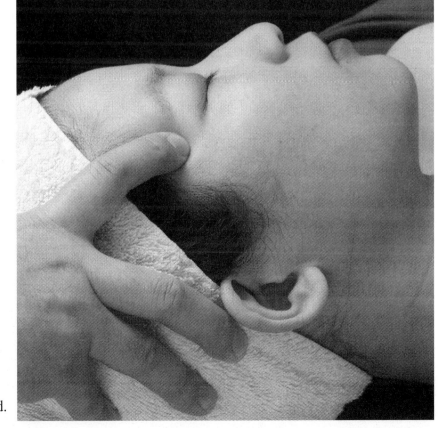

Japanese Facial-Massage Techniques—Example #35

Stroking the *San Sho* Meridian

Japanese name for this technique

二指軽擦法
ni shi kei satsu ho

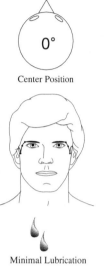

0°

Center Position

Minimal Lubrication

The purpose of this technique

Promote proper *ki* flow on the *San Sho* Meridian

Area of application

Over the temple region along the *San Sho* Meridian

Description

This example demonstrates the procedure of stroking the *San Sho* Meridian. Headaches are often *jitsu* (excessive) conditions; therefore, it is best to sedate *ki* flow of the *San Sho* Meridian by gently stroking in the opposite direction (from outer edge of eyebrow toward the ear) of normal *ki* flow. You can also stroke behind the ear for a good effect. Otherwise, follow the direction of the regular *ki* flow as described.

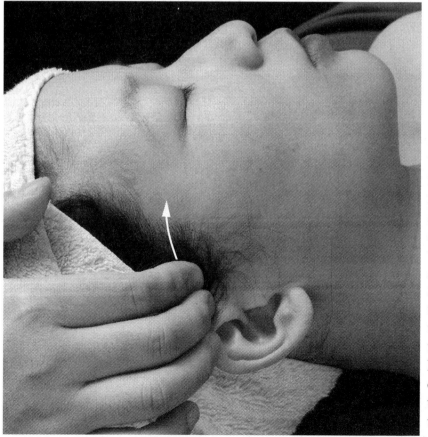

1 Slightly overlap the tips of the index and middle fingers of the right hand. Place the tips of the fingers in the depression just anterior to the upper attachment of the ear where the *ji mon* (*San Sho*-21) is found. Stroke lightly toward the eye until you reach the depression on the temple around the hairline, where you can feel the pulse of the temporal artery at *wa ryo* (*San Sho*-22).

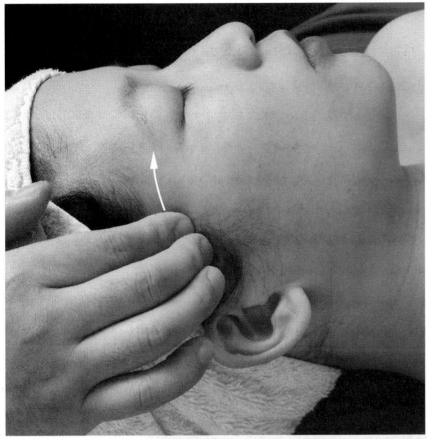

2 Continue the stroke from *wa ryo* (*San Sho*-22), moving toward *shi chiku ku* (*San Sho*-23), which is found in the depression on the lateral edge of the eyebrow.

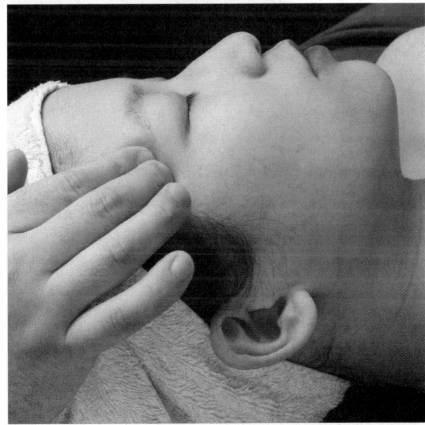

3 End the stroke at *shi chiku ku* (*San Sho*-23). Repeat the sequence two to three times.

Tan Kei—Gall Bladder Meridian

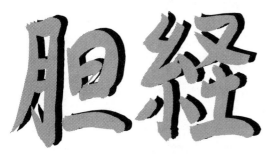

Function of the Gall Bladder Meridian

The main function of the Gall Bladder Meridian is to support the functioning of the Gall Bladder. The Gall Bladder is the only *yang* organ that is not associated with digestion of food and liquid. The Gall Bladder stores the purest liquid of the body (*tan ju*—equivalent to "bile"), and has a close connection to the mental process of decision-making. The Gall Bladder is closely connected to the liver: the two organs work together and affect one another.

Pathway of the Gall Bladder Meridian

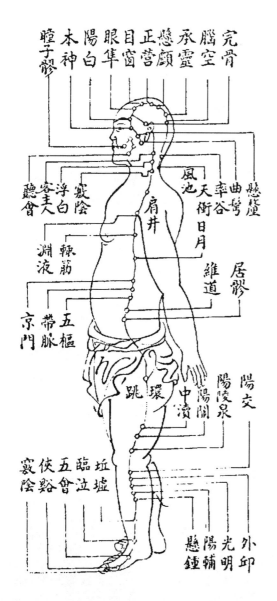

The Gall Bladder Meridian begins at the outer corners of the eyes (Gall Bladder-1) and travels from the front of the ear (Gall Bladder-2) to the upper corner of the hair line (Gall Bladder-4), back behind the ear, and then forward again to the middle of the forehead (Gall Bladder-14). It then runs back over the head and down to the base of the skull (Gall Bladder-20) lateral to the Bladder Meridian. From here it goes to the top of the suprascapula and forward, over the scapula, and along the inside edge of the anterior deltoid.

Next, the Gall Bladder Meridian follows the side of the body with a detour near the end of the Liver Meridian, back across the side of the body to the base of the twelfth rib (Gall Bladder-25, Kidney *bo* Point), then back around the inside of the top of the pelvis bone before angling down the leg, following the lower edge of the gluteus maximus to the side of the leg. Then, the Gall Bladder Meridian follows the lateral side of the leg down to the top of the ankle, running just above the ankle bone and down the top of the foot between the fourth and fifth metatarsals. It ends on the lateral corner of the fourth toe.

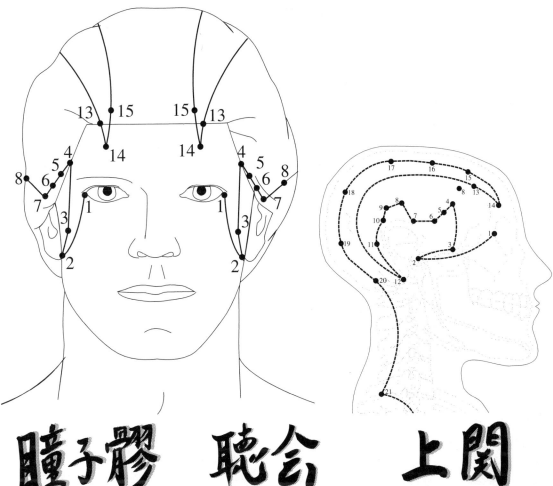

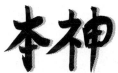

do shi ryo (Gall Bladder-1)
Do means "pupil," *shi* means "son," and *ryo* means "indentation of bone." *Do shi ryo* is used to improve the appearance and remove wrinkles near the lateral edge of eye.

cho e (Gall Bladder-2)
Cho means "to listen" and *e* means "meet" or "gather." It is used to improve the appearance in front of the ear on the side of the cheek. It is also used for tinnitus and jaw tension.

jo kan (Gall Bladder-3)
Jo means "upper" and *kan* means "barrier" or "associate." This *tsubo* is used to reduce muscle tension over the TMJ and improve appearance around this area.

gan en (Gall Bladder-4)
Gan means "chin" and *en* means "rise." When you move the chin (opening the jaw), this point rises on the temple slightly. This *tsubo* is used to improve the appearance around eye and temple region.

hon shin (Gall Bladder-13)
Hon means "origin" or "root" and *shin* means "god" or "emperor." *Hon shin* is used to prevent hair loss at the hairline (especially in the upper corners) and headaches.

yo haku (Gall Bladder-14)
Yo means "yang" or "brightness" and *haku* means "white" or "empty." *Yo haku* is used to improve the appearance of the side of the forehead. It is also used to help relieve headaches and migraines.

Japanese Facial-Massage Techniques—Example #36

Pressure to *Tsubo* on the Gall Bladder Meridian

Japanese name for this technique

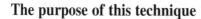

指頭圧迫法

shi to ap paku ho

0°

Center Position

The purpose of this technique

Improve appearance around the lateral edge of the eye

Area of application

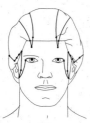

Region from the outside edge of the eye to the temple along the Gall Bladder Meridian

Description

No Lubrication

Ki in the temple region goes out of balance easily, which can cause headaches and migraines. Light stimulation of the facial *tsubo* on the Gall Bladder Meridian helps balance the *ki* of the temple region. This area can be used to balance physical and psychological states of health.

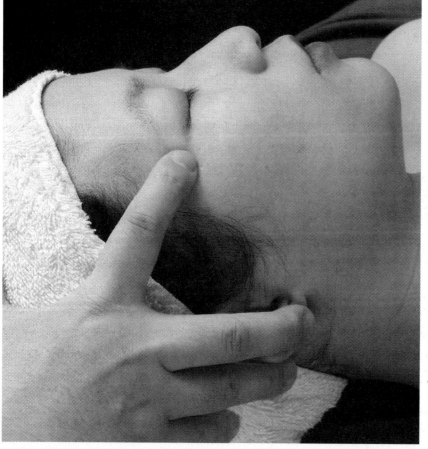

1 Place the thumb, middle, and ring fingers of the right hand on the head to stabilize the hand. Move the position of the supporting fingers as needed to stabilize the hand. Apply light pressure to *do shi ryo* (Gall Bladder-1) with the tip of the index finger. *Do shi ryo* is located in the depression on the bone found at the lateral edge of the eye (at the junction where the zygomatic bone and the frontal eminence bone merge).

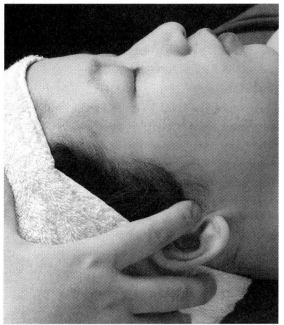

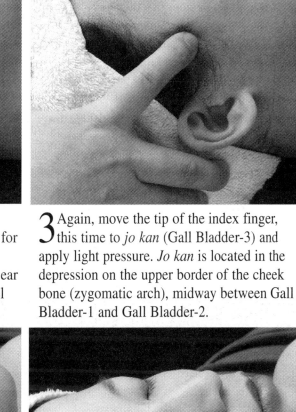

2 Move the tip of the index finger to *cho e* (Gall Bladder-2) and apply light pressure for two to five seconds. *Cho e* is located in the depression in front of the ear lobe where the ear is attached to the face and where you can feel the muscle move when the mouth opens.

3 Again, move the tip of the index finger, this time to *jo kan* (Gall Bladder-3) and apply light pressure. *Jo kan* is located in the depression on the upper border of the cheek bone (zygomatic arch), midway between Gall Bladder-1 and Gall Bladder-2.

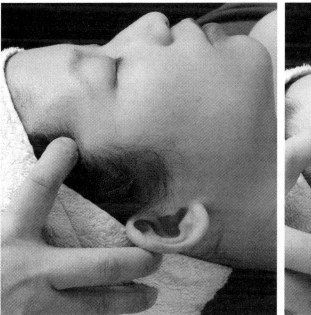

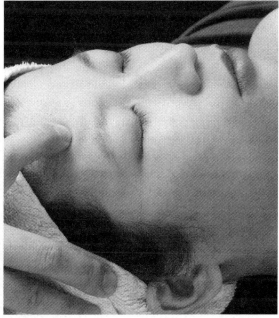

4 Move the tip of the index finger to *gan en* (Gall Bladder-4) and apply light pressure. *Gan en* is located in the depression just behind the temple, slightly into the hairline.

5 Finally, move the tip of the index finger to *yo haku* (Gall Bladder-14) and apply light pressure. Y*o haku* is located in the depression midway between the eyebrow and the hairline directly above the pupil.

Japanese Facial-Massage Techniques—Example #37

Stroking the Gall Bladder Meridian

Japanese name for this technique

二指軽擦法

ni shi kei satsu ho

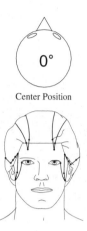

Center Position

Minimal Lubrication

The purpose of this technique

Improve appearance around the lateral edge of the eye

Area of application

Region from the outside edge of the eye to the temple along the Gall Bladder Meridian

Description

The Gall Bladder Meridian has a close relationship to the skin at the edges of the eyes. Stroking this meridian helps prevent or reduce wrinkles around this region. Lubricate sufficiently so that the stroke does not pull the client's skin. Be careful not to get moisturizer or cleanser in the client's hair.

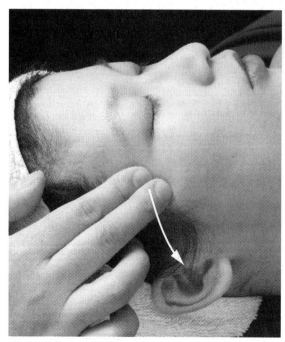

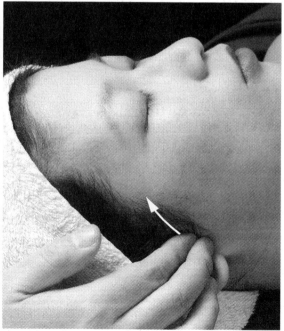

1 Lightly stroke from *do shi ryo* (Gall Bladder-1), found in the depression on the bone found at the lateral edge of the eye toward *cho e* (Gall Bladder-2), found in the depression just in front of the ear lobe where the ear is attached to the face.

2 From *cho e* (Gall Bladder-2), lightly stroke upward along the hairline until you reach *jo kan* (Gall Bladder-3), found in the depression on the upper border of the cheek bone, midway between Gall Bladder-1 and Gall Bladder-2.

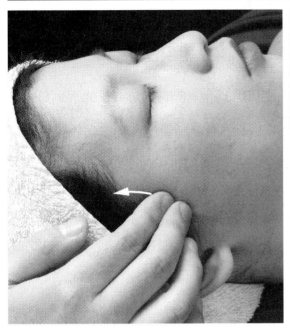

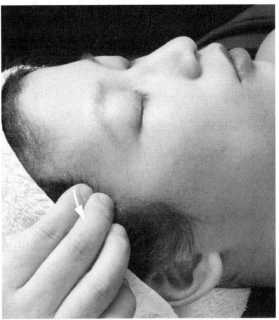

3 Continue stroking from *jo kan* (Gall Bladder-3) until you reach *gan en* (Gall Bladder-4), located in the depression just behind the temple and slightly into the hairline.

4 Once you reach *gan en* (Gall Bladder-4), slightly stroke into the hair. Do not bring too much lubrication into the hair.

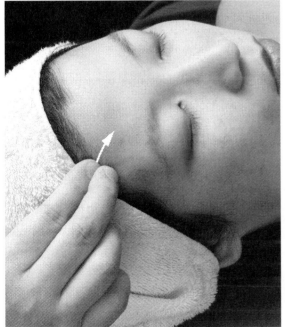

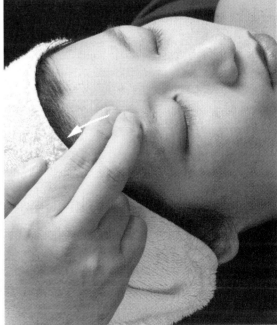

5 Move the fingers to the Gall Bladder Meridian where it returns to the face at the hairline above the eye. Stroke downward toward *yo haku* (Gall Bladder-14), found in the depression midway between the eyebrow and the hairline directly above the pupil.

6 Once you reach *yo haku* (Gall Bladder-14), change the direction of the stroking straight up toward the hairline. Finish the stroke at the hairline. Repeat the entire procedure several times.

Nin Myaku—Conception Vessel

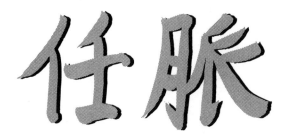

A vessel is different from a meridian: unlike meridians, vessels do not derive directly from particular organs. Vessels divide the body lengthwise, balancing *ki* throughout the body, and maintaining a *ki* balance among the twelve meridians. If a certain part of the body has accumulated too much *ki*, the vessel redistribute it to a section that has become depleted. An unbalanced distribution of *ki* among the meridians generally indicates that the vessels are not functioning properly.

There are eight vessels running across the body. Two of the eight vessels are most commonly used for treatment: *nin myaku* (Conception Vessel) and *toku myaku* (Governing Vessel). Both vessels run along the median line of the body, originating at the anus and terminating inside the mouth, and the twelve meridians run in a symmetrical pattern through the left and right sides of the body on either side of the vessels. These two vessels function primarily to balance *ki* flow in the meridians on the left and right sides of the body.

Function of the Conception Vessel

The primary function of the Conception Vessel is to balance all *yin* meridians. This vessel has a close connection to gynecological problems, including fertility, and regulates the cycles of menstruation.

Pathway of the Conception Vessel

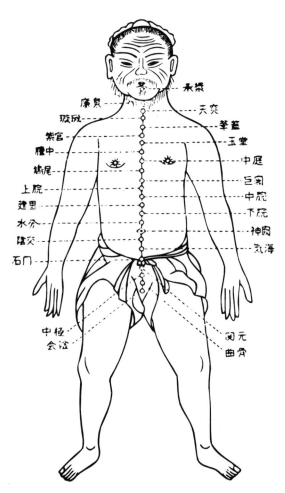

This vessel originates at the anus and travels up the center (median) line of the body to the front of the chin; the last *tsubo* is in the center of the chin, and the vessel continues into the mouth.

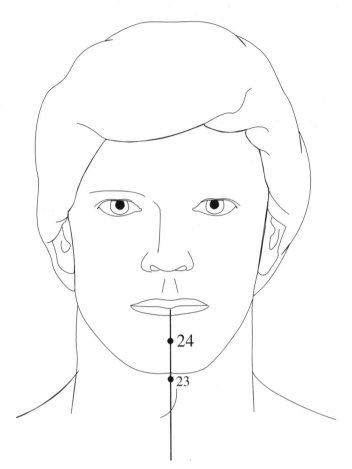

sho sho (Conception Vessel-24)
Sho means "to receive" or "to offer"; the second *sho* means "liquid" or "broth." Together these mean "receiving saliva." *Sho sho* is found in the depression in the center of the chin, midway between the bottom of the lip and the tip of the jaw, directly on the median line. It is often used to improve appearance and reduce muscle tension around the chin. This is also used to treat facial paralysis with acupuncture.

Japanese Facial-Massage Techniques—Example #38

Pressure and Stroking on the Conception Vessel

Japanese names for these techniques

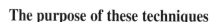

拇指頭圧迫法

bo shi to ap paku ho
ni shi kei satsu ho

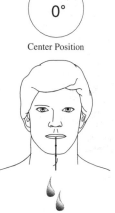

0°

Center Position

The purpose of these techniques

Balancing *ki* flow of the left and right sides of the face

Area of application

Center of the chin on the median line along the Conception Vessel

Description

This technique applies pressure on the *sho sho* (Conception Vessel-24), as explained in Example #15. You can also lightly stroke the Conception Vessel along the neck and under the chin if you desire.

Minimal Lubrication

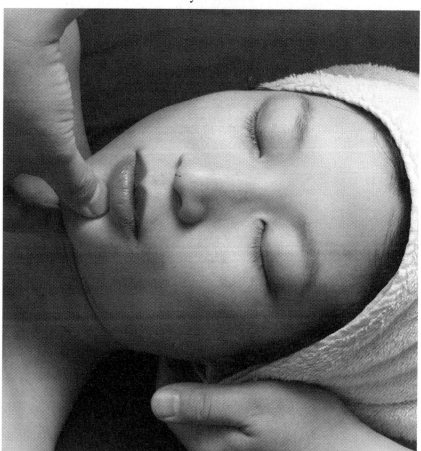

Apply Pressure to Tsubo on the Conception Vessel

1 Place your index, middle, and ring fingers under the clients chin for support. Apply pressure to *sho sho* (Conception Vessel-24) with the tip of your thumb. Hold gentle pressure while the client is exhaling for two to five seconds, then release. This *tsubo* is found in the depression in the center of the chin, midway between the bottom of the lip and the tip of the jaw, directly on the median line.

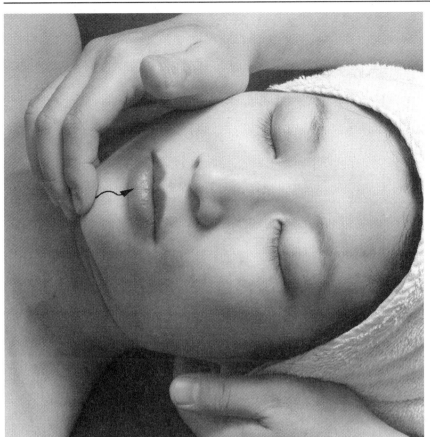

Stroking the Conception Vessel

2 Lightly place the ball of the thumb in front of the ear to stabilize the hand. Place the index finger at the center of the edge of the jawbone. Lightly place the middle finger over the index finger so it slightly overlaps. Slowly stroke along the Conception Vessel toward the lips. Adjust the angle of the wrist according to the contour of the surface.

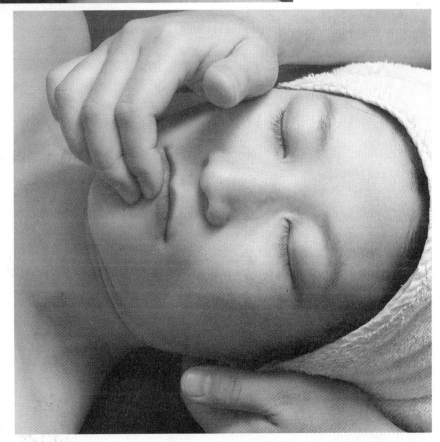

3 End the stroke as you reach the lips. Repeat two to three times.

Toku Myaku—Governing Vessel

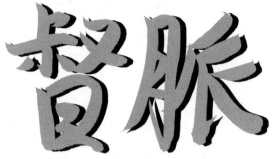

Function of the Governing Vessel

The primary function of the Governing Vessel is to balance the six *yang* meridians. Three *yang* meridians end at the face, and three start at the face. It is very important that the Governing Vessel is working properly to ensure a healthy facial appearance. This vessel governs the functions of the meridians, adjusting them as necessary. This vessel is closely related to the brain, kidneys, spine, central nervous system, and reproductive system.

Irregularity of the Governing Vessel causes diseases in the cranium and kidneys, as well as in the reproductive, digestive, and respiratory systems, and pain in the back and in the neck along the cervical vertebrae.

Pathway of the Governing Vessel

The first point of the Governing Vessel is located at the tip of the coccyx. The Governing Vessel travels up the back along the center of the spine, through the neck, and into the head. Still following the median line, it travels up the back of the head, over the top, and back down the front of the face. The final point is found under the upper lip.

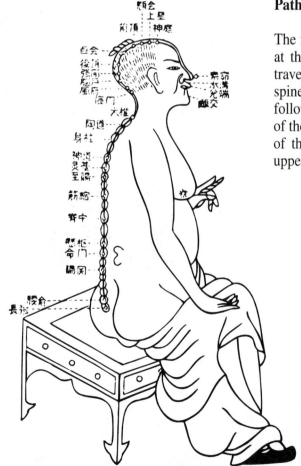

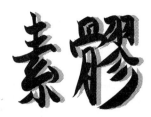

so ryo (Governing Vessel-25)
So means "origin" and *ryo* means "cartilage or bone indentation." Together they mean "common indentation on cartilage." This *tsubo* is found on the small indentation on the cartilage at the tip of the nose. Gentle stimulation of this is used to improve appearance of the entire nose.

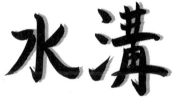

sui ko (Governing Vessel-26)
Sui means "water" or "liquid" and *ko* means "drain." Together they mean "water drains from the nose." This *tsubo* is found midway between the bottom of the tip of the nose and the top edge of the upper lip. It is used to improve appearance between the upper lip and nose and also relieves lumbar pain and epilepsy.

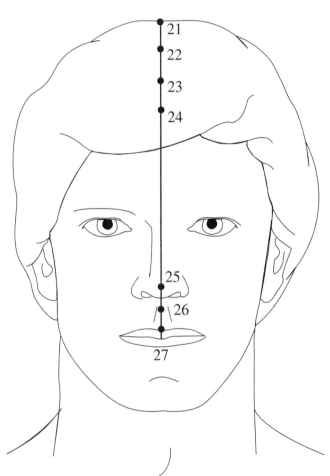

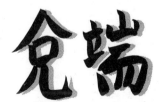

da tan (Governing Vessel-27)
Da means "sharp" and *tan* means "edge." Together they mean "sharp edge of lips." Light stimulation of this *tsubo* is used to improve appearance of the upper lip.

Japanese Facial-Massage Techniques—Example #39

Pressure and Stroking on the Governing Vessel

Japanese names for these techniques

指頭圧迫法

shi to ap paku ho
ni shi kei satsu ho

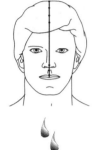

0°

Center Position

The purpose of these techniques

Balancing *ki* flow of the left and right sides of the face

Area of application

Center of the forehead and nose on the median line along the Governing Vessel

Description

Minimal Lubrication

You may need to adjust your pressure according to your client's sensitivity. In general, use only light pressure in this application.

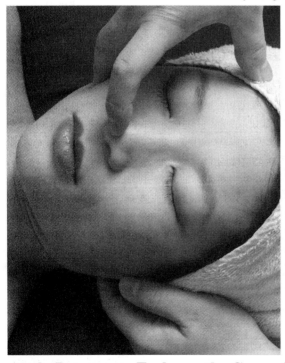

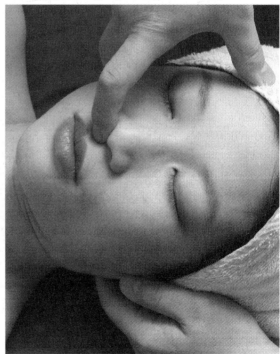

Apply Pressure to Tsubo on the Governing Vessel

1 Place the thumb, middle, and ring fingers to the side of the face to stabilize the hand. Apply light pressure to *so ryo* (Governing Vessel-25) with the tip of your index finger. This *tsubo* is found on the tip of the nose.

2 Move the index finger to *sui ko* (Governing Vessel-26) and apply light pressure. *Sui ko* is found midway between the bottom tip of the nose and the top edge of the upper lip.

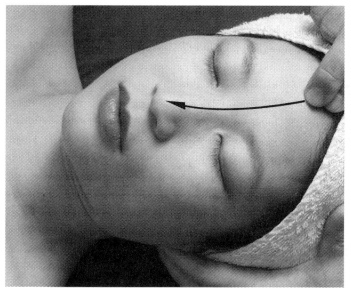

Stroking the Governing Vessel

3 Gently support the side of the head with your left hand. Place the overlapping index and middle fingers of the right hand onto the center of the forehead by the hairline. Start stroking down the middle of the face across the forehead, between the eyebrows, and down the center of the nose to the tip where you find *so ryo* (Governing Vessel-25). Keep the stroking very gentle, especially on the top of the nose.

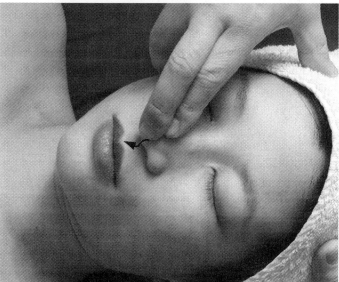

4 Slide down along the nose toward the lips to *sui ko* (Governing Vessel-26).

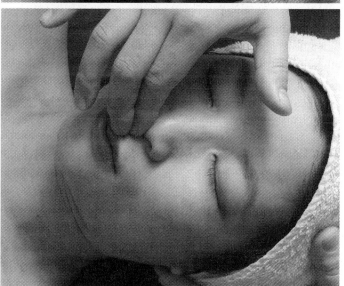

5 Continue stroking until you reach the upper edge of the lips and then stop. Repeat several times as desired. Do not stroke into the lips or mouth.

Japanese Facial-Massage Techniques—Example #40

Pressure on *In Do* (Third Eye Region)

Japanese name for this technique

指頭圧迫法

shi to ap paku ho

Center Position

The purpose of this technique

Balance and promote the *ki* flow of the entire face

Area of application

Just above the center point between the two eyebrows

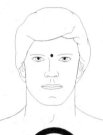

Description

This technique finishes the energizing stage of Japanese facial massage by applying pressure on *in do* or *san me*, also known as the third eye. This *tsubo* is *ki ketsu*, an extraordinary point. It appears to be on the Governing Vessel, and although the location is on the Governing Vessel, it does not actually belong to it.

No Lubrication

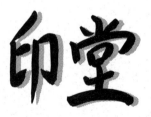

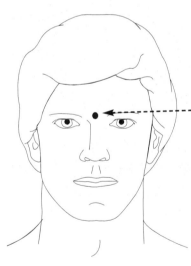

- - - - - *in do* (extraordinary point)

In means "stamp" or "mark" and *do* means "house" or "temple." This *tsubo* is also called *san me* (*san* means "three" or "third" and *me* means "eye") and is known as the third eye. This is one of the most well-known *ki ketsu* (extraordinary *tsubo*) and is known as the indicator for one's physical and psychological conditions. The location of *in do* is often confused with that of *gan chu* (another extraordinary *tsubo*), which is located just above *in do*. The *in do* is located in the bone depression between the eyebrows on median line of the face. Traditionally, this *tsubo* is known to calm people who experience psychological oversensitivity, and it is especially used with hypertraumatic children. *In do* is often used in Japanese facial massage to help calm the client and balance the *ki* flow throughout the face. It has a very close relation with lack of color in the face; light stimulation helps refresh a pallid complexion. Traditionally, one is always taught to press *in do* with the middle finger. Pressure on this *tsubo* also helps balance physical and emotional conditions.

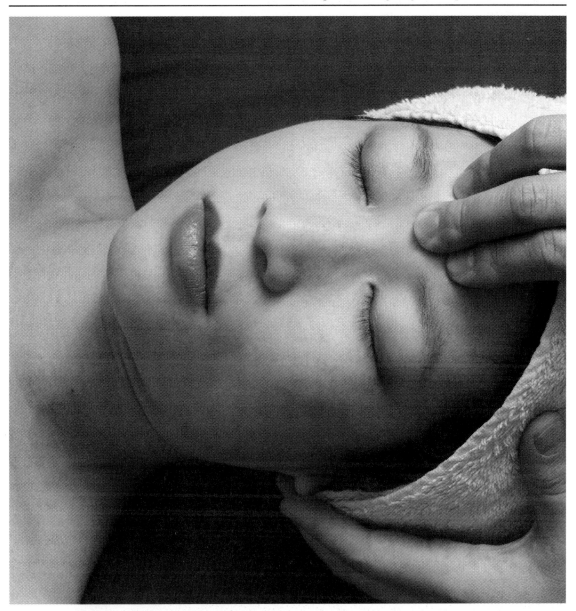

1 Place the index, middle, and ring fingers of your hand together, using the index and ring fingers to stabilize the middle finger. Place the middle finger in the *in do*, between the eyebrows and slightly up into the forehead.

2 Apply pressure to *in do*. The pressure should be maintained for thirty seconds to one minute, or as long as you desire.

Chapter Ten

FINISHING TOUCH

In this chapter, I explain five examples of the techniques used to offer a smooth finish to a facial massage. Massage is like music in that you know when the song is coming to an end. Through these massage techniques, the client will sense when the end of the massage is near, and this is better than hearing a verbal message from the therapist. Generally I end my facial massages with slow, smooth movements, preferring a very relaxed finish to the entire session. This is the same as with a full-body massage. The slowing of the tempo toward the end of the massage is a very important signal to the client's body and mind that the massage is coming to an end.

After the full-facial massage, the face will have collected toxins and gasses which have been released from the muscle tissue. The purpose of the finishing touch procedure is to drain this unwanted matter from the face into the body's lymphatic system where it is flushed out naturally. To maximize the effects of the Japanese facial massage, this is an important procedure to perform at the end so the toxins do not remain in the facial regions.

To drain the accumulated toxins into the lymphatic system, apply very light strokes evenly over the facial surface. Excessive pressure blocks the movement of fluid, and the toxins will not drain properly. The speed of the stroke must be very slow—about five to ten seconds per inch. A slow stroke is necessary to work with the lymphatic system—if you stroke faster, fluid in the lymphatic system is unable to move, rendering the technique ineffective.

As with any form of body massage, it is important to encourage your client to drink water plentifully (at least one liter) shortly after the massage is completed.

Japanese Facial-Massage Techniques—Example #41

Slow Stroking up the Side of the Face

Japanese name for this technique

Center Position

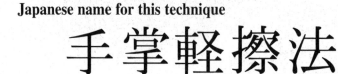

shu sho kei satsu ho

The purpose of this technique

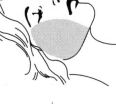

Redistribute the lubrication

Area of application

From the sides of the cheeks to the temple region

Description

Generous Lubrication

Start the finishing-touch procedures with this technique to redistribute the moisturizer to the sides of the cheeks. During the energizing stage, the side of the face is often unevenly lubricated, and this technique ensures that the side of the face is evenly lubricated once again. If the face is dry, add just enough lubrication to allow smooth stroking without pulling the skin. This technique applies slight tension to reawaken the muscles over the cheeks to help with the final stage of facial massage.

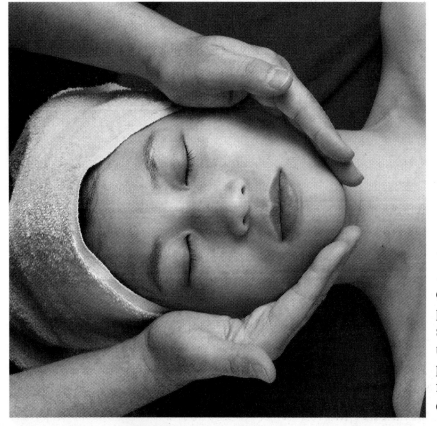

1 For this technique, cup the client's cheeks with your palms. The fingers should gently wrap under the chin. Your palms should be floating freely, directly over the ears.

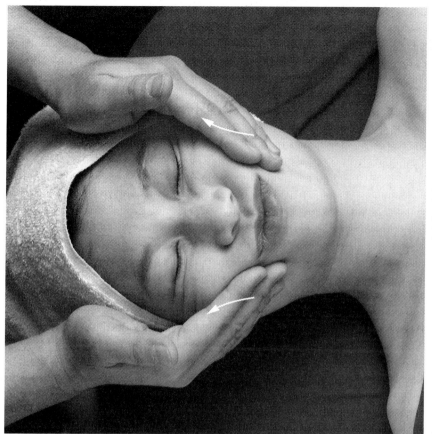

2 Start stroking over the cheek with medium pressure so the facial skin lightly gathers over the cheekbone. Slightly bend your palms to adjust to the contours of the cheeks. Slowly release the pressure on the cheeks and slide your fingers toward the temple region.

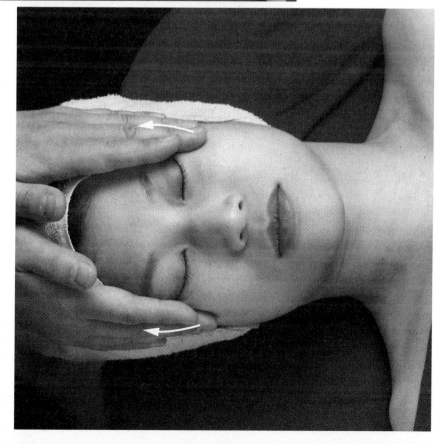

3 Continue stroking up over the temple region to the edge of the forehead and gently release your hands from the face. Repeat the entire procedure several times.

Japanese Facial-Massage Techniques—Example #42

Stroking the Forehead with the Thumbs

Japanese name for this technique

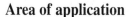

拇指軽擦法

bo shi kei satsu ho

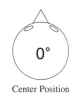

0°

Center Position

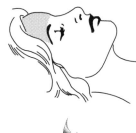

Minimal Lubrication

The purpose of this technique

Drain the toxins in the lymphatic system, from the forehead to the cheek

Area of application

The forehead

Description

The next three examples demonstrate lymphatic-drainage techniques for the face and the neck. When you are trying to drain the toxins from the lymphatic system, you must work on the surface layer of the skin. Pressure must be kept as light as possible, and you must keep your strokes very slow. The lymphatic system cannot move when you are using faster strokes.

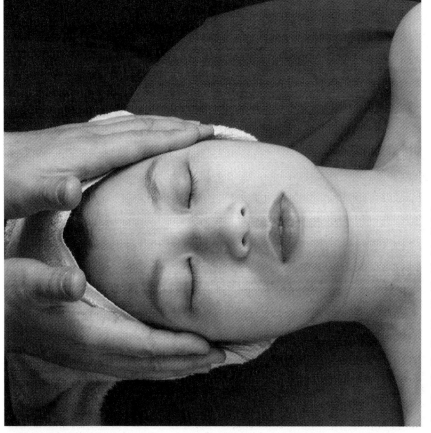

1 With the client's head in the center position, place the tips of your index and middle fingers at the temple regions, using the same starting positions as in the last technique. However, drop your wrists slightly so bases of the thumbs almost contact the top of head.

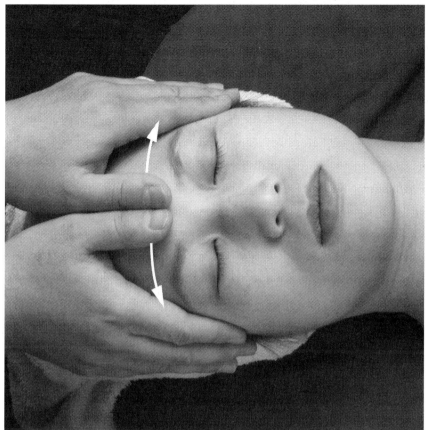

2 Place the sides of your thumbs together in the middle of the forehead with the thumbtips pointed toward the nose. Apply very light, even pressure, and spread the thumbs laterally toward the temples. Keep your fingertips anchored and stroke slowly.

3 Use the entire length of the sides of the thumbs for this stroke, keeping the phalanges contoured against the forehead. Your thumbs should remain parallel throughout, moving from the center out toward the fingers on each side of the head. Cover the entire forehead. Repeat two to three.

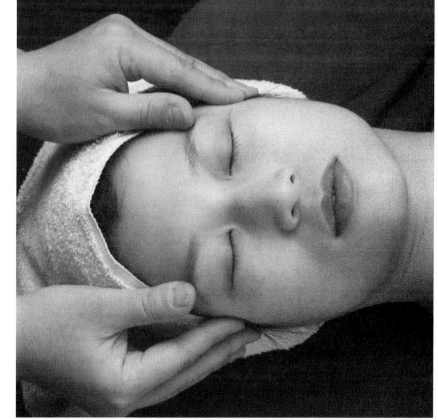

Japanese Facial-Massage Techniques—Example #43

Thumb Stroking down the Side of the Face

Japanese name for this technique

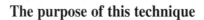

拇指軽擦法

bo shi kei satsu ho

0°

Center Position

The purpose of this technique

Drain the toxins through the lymphatic system, from the face to the neck

Area of application

On the masseter and the cheeks between the cheekbone and jaw

Description

This example continues the draining of toxins from the lymphatic system. This procedure can be done with one thumb, but it is more often performed with two (both techniques are demonstrated here). This technique is usually applied with the client's head in the center position. As needed, you can turn the head slightly for better access to the right cheek.

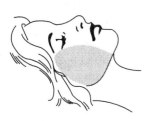

Minimal Lubrication

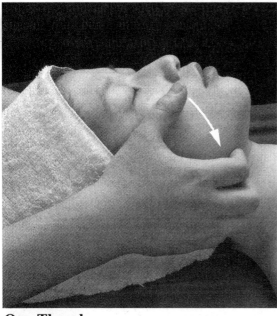

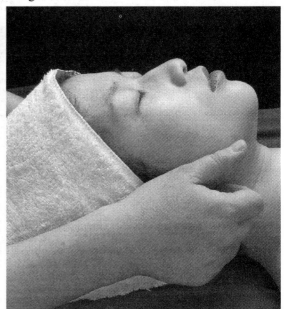

One Thumb

1 Lightly place the tips of your index and middle fingers under the jaw. Gently place the entire side of thumb directly over the cheek bone, just below the eye. Slowly stroke over the cheek with the thumb, toward the index finger.

2 As the thumb reaches the edge of the jaw, stop and repeat. As you continue to stroke, you can move the thumb in either direction, toward the nose or ear to cover the entire cheek region.

Both Thumbs

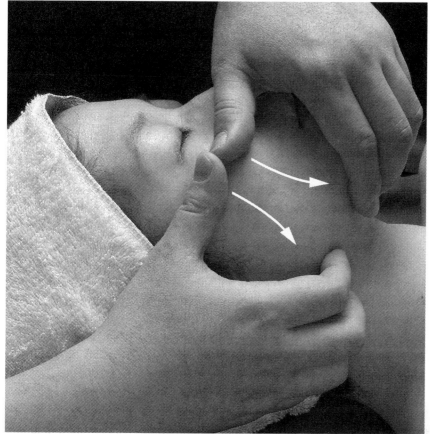

3 This is similar to stroking with one thumb, but instead uses both thumbs together. Maintain the starting position as shown in Step 1 for the right hand. Place the tip of the index and middle fingers of your left hand under the jaw near the chin. Place the thumb of your left hand just below the eye, next to the right thumb. The thumbs should slightly overlap. Slowly stroke down the cheek toward the jaw with both thumbs together.

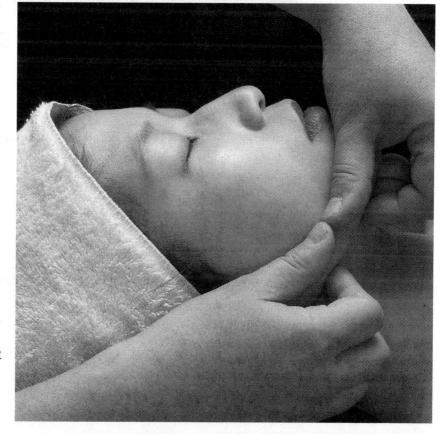

4 As the thumbs reach the edge of the jaw, stop stroking. Keep the strokes very light and slow. Repeat five to ten times as needed, then repeat on the other cheek.

Japanese Facial-Massage Techniques—Example #44

Light Stroking down the Front of the Neck

Japanese name for this technique

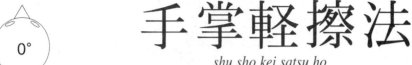

shu sho kei satsu ho

Center Position

The purpose of this technique

Drain the toxins through the lymphatic system, from the neck to the rest of the body

Area of application

Front of the neck and the clavicle area

Description

This is the final stage of lymphatic drainage, which flushes the toxins from the neck down to the rest of the body. It takes some practice to apply smoothly, with light, even pressure. It is important for your elbows and shoulders to remain relaxed.

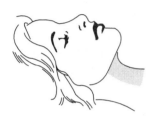

Minimal Lubrication

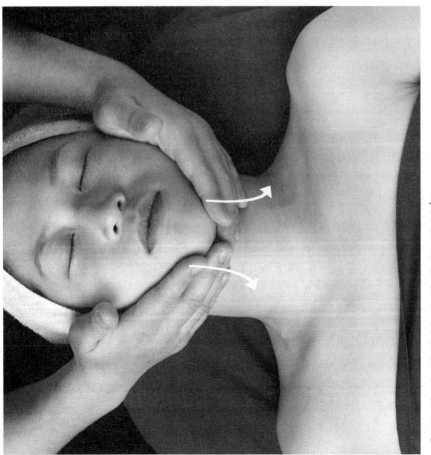

1 Place your fingers under the client's jaw, with the palms in front of the ears. Do not apply any pressure into the face. Start slowly stroking down the front of the neck toward the body. If the neck is dry, add a minimal amount of lubrication. Do not use excessive lubrication—use only enough so your hands slide easily down the neck.

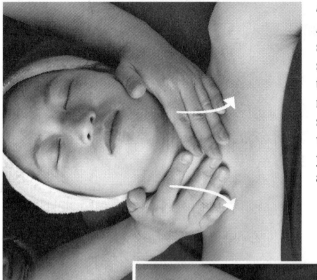

2 Continue slowly stroking down the neck as lightly as possible. All fingers should be relaxed to fit the contours and shape of the neck. The fingertips should touch slightly so the hands cover the entire neck. Your palms should lightly touch the sides of the neck while stroking. With your wrists remaining loose, stroke by moving your hands from the elbows and shoulders and not just by rotating the wrists.

3 Continue to stroke down the neck. Once you reach the crook of the neck, rotate your wrists and change the direction of the stroke toward the client's shoulders. The fingers should stroke across the upper chest and over the collar (clavicle) bone.

4 Once you reach the shoulders, let your hands gently slide off the edges. Repeat this entire procedure several times.

Japanese Facial-Massage Techniques—Example #45

Light Two-Finger Pressure over Closed Eyes

Japanese name for this technique

二指圧迫法

ni shi ap paku ho

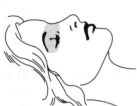

0°

Center Position

The purpose of this technique

Relax the client

Area of application

On top of closed eyes

Description

Finish the Japanese facial massage by applying extremely light finger pressure on the closed eyes. This provides a relaxing moment for you and the client as the treatment is concluded.

It is best if the client is not wearing contact lenses when you apply this technique. If they are wearing lenses, you can avoid this technique entirely.

No Lubrication

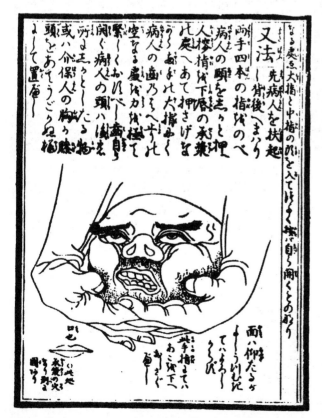

Centuries-old Japanese facial-massage text

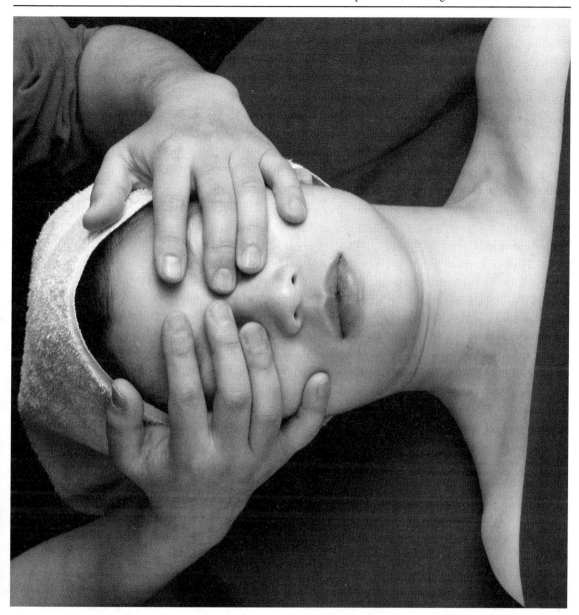

1 Lightly rest your palms over the client's ears, relaxing your elbows and shoulders. Gently place your middle and ring fingers over the closed eyes. Release all tension in your hands, and allow your fingers to drop lightly down to the face. You can use the index and middle fingers instead, but the combination of middle and ring fingers generally fits the contour of the eyes well and provides more gentle pressure.

2 **Do not apply any downward pressure with your fingers.** Hold for fifteen to thirty seconds or as long as you desire. Gently release the pressure and remove your hands.

FINAL THOUGHTS

Beauty and youthfulness are desirable to women and men across the world. We all possess these traits early in our lives, but when they begin to fade, what can we do? There are many products and massage methods in the world which claim to address this problem effectively, but how many of these products or methods actually do what they claim? One thing is for certain: there is no natural procedure which produces instant results. Beauty and youthfulness are the reflection of optimal health; health is the important beginning. Japanese facial massage (especially in combination with other Japanese health modalities) nourishes health, which is then radiated as beauty.

In your decision to learn Japanese facial massage, you are undertaking the most refined and effective facial-therapy system in existence. Japanese facial massage is a traditional Japanese art, like tea ceremony or calligraphy, and has a long history, with countless additions and refinements made by generations of masters. Great effort has gone into perfecting this therapy.

In Japan, there is great respect for the traditional arts—it is common knowledge that a practitioner goes through deep training to gain experience and skill to deliver a competent performance. When a practitioner is finally able to give such a performance, it is certain to be of a profound and moving nature: the training guarantees it. Without this training, the performance is not authentic; it may seem similar, but it is obviously not the genuine thing and is devoid of real substance. To serve green tea in a Japanese cup is nice, but it is not an authentic tea ceremony; when an amateur writes a character with brush and ink, it may be pretty, but it is certainly not true calligraphy. Similarly, merely using Japanese facial-massage techniques does not ensure the benefits of Japanese facial massage. Any traditional art takes significant time to master, and when this time is invested, one learns the art in a genuine way. It is only a matter of dedication.

Traditionally, one learns this art along with the daily practice of traditional Japanese meditation (*zazen*—Zen meditation). What develops from this is a total sensitization and relaxation of mind and body which is referred to as "centeredness." When mind and body are unified in this way, one can give massage therapy with a degree of confidence and awareness unreachable by massage training alone. Do not overlook meditation training (*zazen*, *shamatha*, and *vipashyana* are all appropriate traditional forms of meditation that are taught widely). Meditation enhances your practice when you are beginning, and it is essential for the advanced-level practitioner.

At the most advanced levels, Japanese facial massage is a deep subject. It becomes necessary to understand the concepts on which the advanced Japanese facial-massage techniques are built. Traditional Japanese medical concepts such as *Yin/Yang* Theory and Five Element Theory, *keiraku*, and *tsubo* must be learned along with the connections and correlation to one another. Also, one must understand traditional Japanese facial diagnosis, which is an essential skill for professional-level practice. Finally, one must understand clinical study to treat various facial problems and make extremely fine adjustments in core techniques to treat individual facial conditions properly.

I have tried very hard to describe Japanese facial massage accurately, but there are limitations to studying massage from a book, regardless of the number of photographs and illustrations. Massage is a subtle art beyond the reach of words. Since it is not possible for me to be with all students interested in learning Japanese facial massage, this book can serve as a reference during the preliminary stage of study.

As a practitioner of this art, it is important to understand all aspects of the massage techniques. It is best to learn with a partner so you can receive the same massage techniques you are learning. Your partner becomes a crucial touchstone throughout the educational process, and you should give each other straightforward criticism. When you know how each technique affects your face and when you are familiar with the varieties of pressure contained within the facial-massage repertoire, you will be ready to give excellent facial therapy.

This book is the popular edition of the Professional Facial Massage training manual. I have drawn the core facial-massage techniques from the professional edition and offered them here so that the student can learn the essential techniques alone. Also I have developed a video-tape to supplement this book. If you are interested in this, or in further training, or if you have any questions, comments or suggestions about the material covered in this book, or if you want information about my

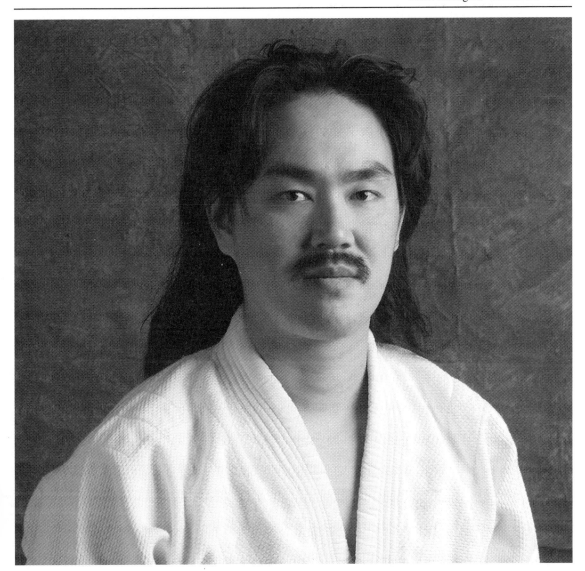

workshops, feel free to contact me. Thanks again to all those people who show interest in our way of healing.

Good health to you!

Shogo Mochizuki

c/o Kotobuki Publications
P.O. Box 19917
Boulder, CO   80308-2917
www.japanesemassage.org

INDEX

BIBLIOGRAPHY

Anatomical References

Clemente, Carmine D. *Anatomy: A Regional Atlas of the Human Body*.
3rd ed. Munich: Urban & Schwarzenberg, 1987.

Rohen, Johannes W. and Yokochi, Chihiro. *Color Atlas of Anatomy*.
2nd ed. New York: Igaku-Shoin, 1988.

Acupuncture Point Reference

Kinoshita, Haruto. *Illustration of Acupuncture Point*.
21st ed. Tokyo: Ido No Nippon Sha, 1995.

JAPANESE FACIAL MASSAGE QUICK REFERENCES

Massage Techniques for the Neck

Example #1. Up-Stroking on the Side of the Neck
Example #2. Light Stroking up the Front of the Neck
Example #3. Stroking under the Chin
Example #4. Paddle Percussion under the Chin
Example #5. Light Stroking up the Side of the Neck

Basic Japanese Facial-Massage Techniques

Example #6. Stroking up the Side of the Face
Example #7. Stroking up the Side of the Face with Both Hands
Example #8. Flip-Stroking on the Jawbone with the Thumb
Example #9. Two-Finger Walking on the Cheeks
Example #10. Combination Stroking over the Edge of the Jaw
Example #11. Flip-Stroking on the Top of the Cheekbone
Example #12. Combination Stroking on Top of the Cheekbone
Example #13. Light Stroking up the Cheek with Two Fingers
Example #14. Kneading the Chin with the Thumbs
Example #15. Pressure and Rotation on the Center of the Chin
Example #16. Thumb Pressure on the Lower Face
Example #17. Kneading the Forehead with the Thumbs
Example #18. Stroking on the Forehead with the Thumbs
Example #19. Light Percussion on the Face with Four Fingers
Example #20. Finger Stroking on the Side of the Nose
Example #21. Circular Stroking on the Side of the Nose
Example #22. Stroking on the Nose
Example #23. Stroking the Lips
Example #24. Stroking in Front of the Ear
Example #25. Circular Stroking around the Eyes

Energizing Techniques

Example #26. Pressure to *Tsubo* on the Large Intestine Meridian
Example #27. Stroking the Large Intestine Meridian
Example #28. Pressure to *Tsubo* on the Stomach Meridian
Example #29. Stroking the Stomach Meridian
Example #30. Pressure to *Tsubo* on the Small Intestine Meridian
Example #31. Stroking the Small Intestine Meridian
Example #32. Pressure to *Tsubo* on the Bladder Meridian
Example #33. Stroking the Bladder Meridian
Example #34. Pressure to *Tsubo* on the *San Sho* Meridian
Example #35. Stroking the *San Sho* Meridian
Example #36. Pressure to *Tsubo* on the Gall Bladder Meridian
Example #37. Stroking the Gall Bladder Meridian
Example #38. Pressure and Stroking on the Conception Vessel
Example #39. Pressure and Stroking on the Governing Vessel
Example #40. Pressure on *In Do* (Third Eye Region)

Finishing Touch

Example #41. Slow Stroking up the Side of the Face
Example #42. Stroking the Forehead with the Palms
Example #43. Thumb Stroking down the Side of the Face
Example #44. Light Stroking down the Front of the Neck
Example #45. Light Two-Finger Pressure over Closed Eyes

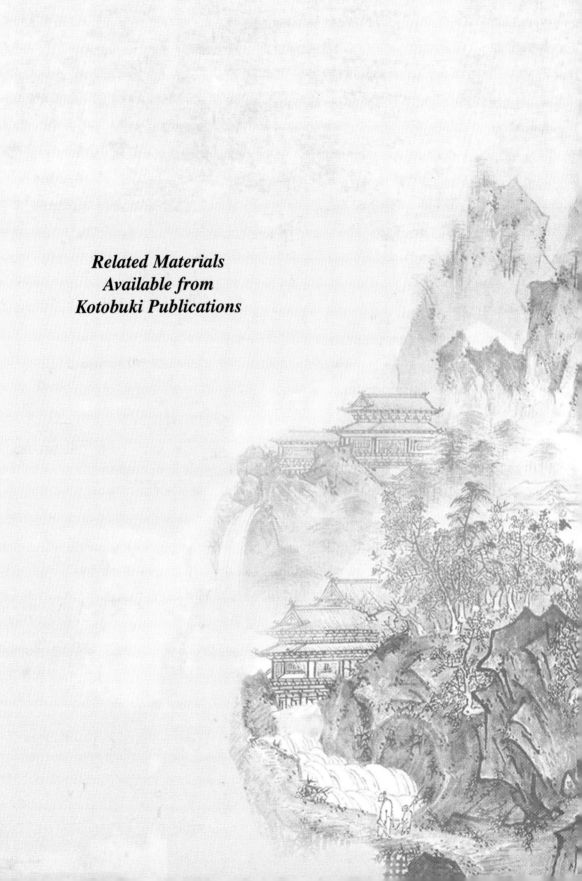

Related Materials
Available from
Kotobuki Publications

Kotobuki Popular Editions

The popular editions have been extracted from the professional editions of our publications. We have selected easy-to-learn techniques that give step-by-step instructions for laypeople, massage therapists and students, and various health professionals. We have also minimized the professional anatomical and medical terminology so anyone can enjoy and benefit from the popular editions. Videos are available to supplement the textbooks as visual aids, and they demonstrate all examples in the textbooks. However, the videos do not contain basic, important information, such as the precautions, set-up procedures, and concepts. The videos are created specifically to act as a visual supplementation for use with the textbooks, and therefore are not sold independently (call for information).

Ko Bi Do™ : The Art of Japanese Facial Massage
Popular Edition

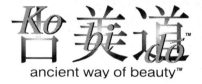

ancient way of beauty™

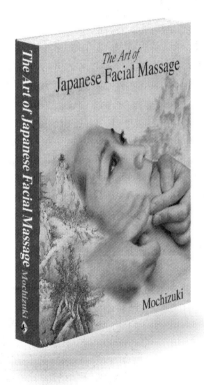

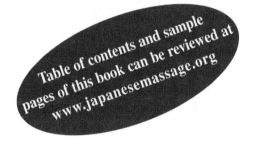

Table of contents and sample pages of this book can be reviewed at www.japanesemassage.org

This book features:

- Application techniques of Japanese facial massage
- Japanese concepts of health and beauty
- 45 examples for the face and neck
- Over 300 detailed photos and illustrations
- 187 pgs softcover, ISBN 1-57615-053-4

Book only $ 19.⁹⁵

Japanese facial massage is different from every other method of facial massage. It uniquely combines the very effective methods of facial massage with traditional East Asian concepts. Forty-five examples of techniques covering the face and neck are demonstrated throughout the three different stages of application. Over 300 photographs and illustrations supplement over 187 pages of detailed text.

Ko bi do™: Ancient Way of Beauty
The Art of Japanese Facial Massage
Book & Video Set

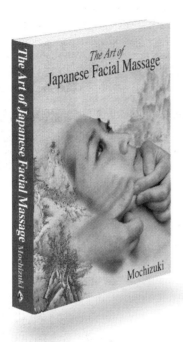
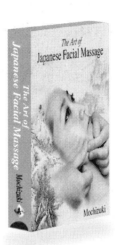

This video supplements the popular edition of *The Art of Japanese Facial Massage* with vivid demonstrations of each of the forty-five easy-to-learn examples found in the textbook. It also demonstrates how to combine the techniques to construct a full-facial massage. All demonstrations are done by Shogo Mochizuki.

This video features:

- Basic facial massage application techniques
- 45 application examples for the face and neck
- Demonstration of three stage facial massage treatment
- Approx. 60 minutes running time.
- ISBN 1-57615-054-2

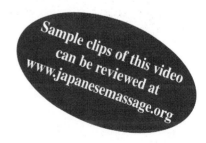

Sample clips of this video can be reviewed at www.japanesemassage.org

Book and Video set   ISBN 1-57615-055-0 $ 59.⁹⁰

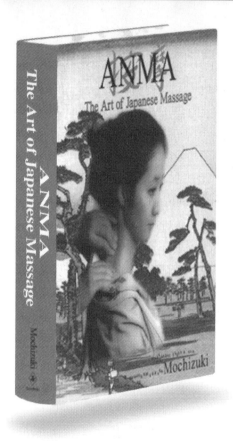
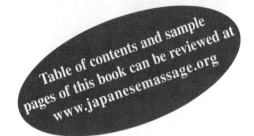
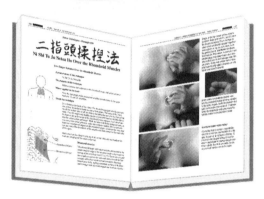

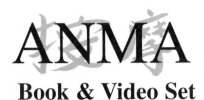

ANMA
Book & Video Set

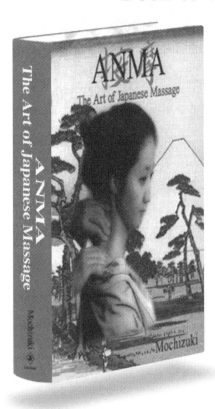
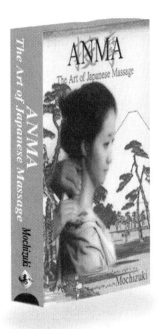

This video supplements the popular edition of *Anma: The Art of Japanese Massage*. It demonstrates forty-five easy-to-learn examples and visually supplements the textbook. It also demonstrates how to combine the techniques to construct a smooth, therapeutic full-body massage. Demonstrated by Shogo Mochizuki.

This video features:

- Nine anma application techniques
- 45 application examples for the entire body
- Approx. 60 minutes running time
- ISBN 1-57615-051-8

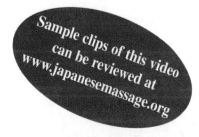

Sample clips of this video can be reviewed at www.japanesemassage.org

Book and Video set   ISBN 1-57615-052-6 $ 59.^{90}

Kotobuki Popular Editions

Zoku Shin Do™
The Art of Japanese Foot Massage
Popular Edition

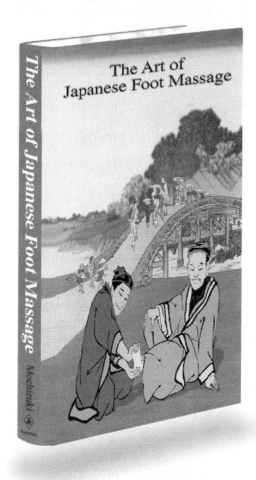

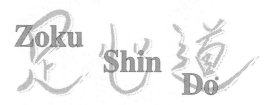

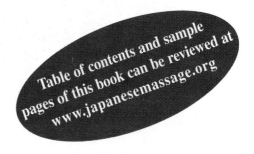

Table of contents and sample pages of this book can be reviewed at www.japanesemassage.org

This book features:
- Application techniques of Japanese foot massage
- Brief history and principles of zoku shin do
- 45 examples of applications for the foot
- Over 300 detailed photos and illustrations
- 191 pgs softcover, ISBN 1-57615-056-9
  $ 19.^{95}

Zoku shin do, the oldest known form of East Asian foot reflexology, originated in China over five thousand years ago. **The Art of Japanese Foot Massage** explains the method of foot massage that arose from this ancient tradition. Forty-five easy-to-follow examples of foot-massage techniques are shown. This book also includes detailed explanations of meridians and pressure points. Over 300 photographs and illustrations span this 191-page volume.

Zoku Shin Do™
The Art of Japanese Foot Massage
Book & Video Set

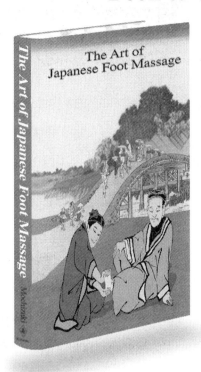
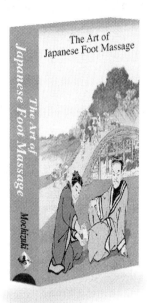

This video supplements the text of *The Art of Japanese Foot Massage*. It demonstrates all forty-five easy-to-learn examples found in the textbook. It also demonstrates how to combine these techniques seamlessly to construct a therapeutic foot massage. Demonstrated by Shogo Mochizuki.

This video features:

- Basic foot application techniques
- 45 application examples for the foot
- Demonstrates how to combine techniques
- Approx. 60 minutes running time
- ISBN 1-57615-057-7

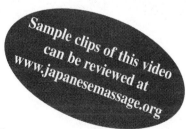

Sample clips of this video can be reviewed at www.japanesemassage.org

Book and Video set   ISBN 1-57615-058-5 $ 59.^{90}

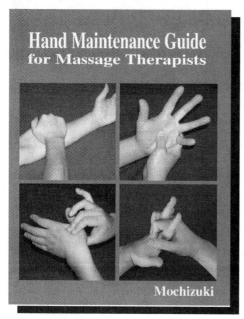
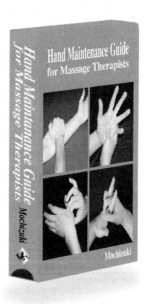

Ko Bi Do™ : The Art of Japanese Facial Massage
Professional Edition

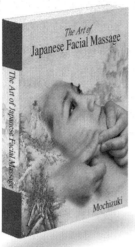

Japanese facial massage is one of the most effective methods for the prevention and treatment of wrinkles and age spots. Never before has a more extensive book been published on this subject! A combination of traditional concepts and more modern techniques have been brought together to provide a fresh approach to the professional beauty and massage industry.

This book features:
- Application techniques of Japanese facial massage
- Japanese concepts of health and beauty
- 65 examples for the face and neck
- Over 600 detailed photos and illustrations
- ISBN 1-57615-093-3

Zoku Shin Do® Foot Reflexology
Professional Edition

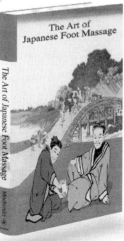

An in depth study of the foot massage portion of Zoku Shin Do and over a hundred examples and techniques are provided in this book. Included are techniques for use in both the supine and prone positions. Over a thousand illustrations and pictures will walk you through the techniques that you need to know to give a very effective foot massage at a professional level.

This book features:
- Application techniques of Japanese foot massage
- Brief history and principles of zoku shin do
- 110 examples of applications for the foot
- Over 1,000 detailed photos and illustrations
- softcover, ISBN 1-57615-096-8

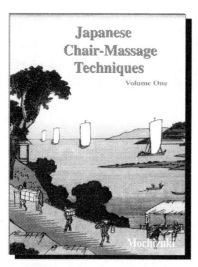
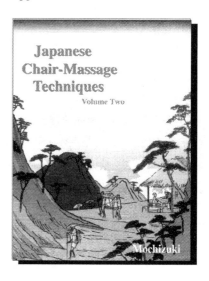

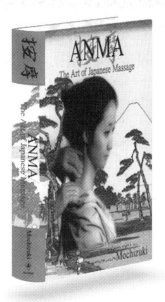
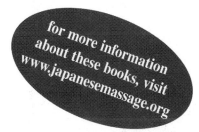
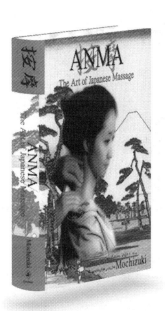

Japanese Massage Intensive Workshops

The Japanese Massage and Bodywork Institute in Boulder, Colorado offers intensive workshops several times each year. Also, smaller seminars are available throughout the United States, and also in Europe and Brazil. For information and dates of these programs, call us or visit our website.

ANMA: The Art of Japanese Massage Certification Course

Koho anma is the therapeutic core of anma practice. Our classes combine *koho* anma (traditional anma) and *genko* anma (modern anma). Ninety percent of this course will involve hands-on training, but there will also be an introduction to North East Asian medical theory including tsubo, meridian theory and diagnosis. This is a rare opportunity to study directly with one of the most experienced and knowledgeable anma instructors/practitioners.

Japanese Chair-Massage Techniques Certification Course

Chair Massage is the fastest growing adjunct modality for massage therapists. After seven years of development, drawing from an extensive repertorie of both anma and shiatsu, Mochizuki has developed this modality to bring chair massage to its highest therapeutic potential. Ninety percent of this course will involve hands-on training. These arts are best suited for chair massage for they are non-oil based and applied over clothing, which is typical to chair massage. This course will be supported by and draw upon the most thorough textbooks within the art.

The Art of Japanese Facial Massage
Certification Course

Japanese Facial Massage is different from every other method of facial massage. It uniquely combines modern methods of facial massage with traditional East Asian concepts. Japanese facial massage techniques originated in anma, and were further refined in the field of cosmetology to effectively work on the face. They are performed very lightly with smooth stroking and quick, light, percussive techniques. The stimulation is not heavy, but it affects the underlying tissues to increase the blood circulation, enhance the condition of the skin and minimize the aging process.

In this course you will learn:
- Three stages of facial massage treatment: cleansing, moisturizing, and energizing
- Basic and advanced facial technique
- Neck and shoulder massage
- Descriptions and locations of keiraku (meridians) and tsubo (acupoints) on the face
- Facelift technique using tsubo (acupoint) and meridians
- Masque and exfoliation
- Product selection for various skin types
- Basic Japanese foot massage

Zoku Shin Do® Reflexology
Certification Course

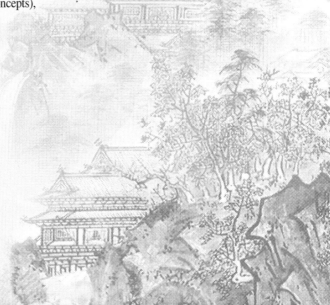

Zoku Shin Do (Traditional East Asian Foot Reflexology), is the oldest known form of reflexology, having originated in China over five thousand years ago. Zoku Shin Do uniquely combines foot massage, *Keiraku* (meridian concepts), Tsubo (acupoints), *Zo Fu Hansha* (internal organ reflection), and *Keiraku Hansha* (meridian reflection theory) to balance the physical and psychological aspects of the client. It is based on the *Yin/Yang*, Five Elements, and Meridian theorem, rather than the Zone Theory of Western Reflexology. The foot is the foundation of the body's structure and health. Japanese foot massage combines very fast, light, and smooth techniques along with slow, deep, stimulating techniques to enhance the client's health. It was originally developed by Zoku Shin Do practitioners as a warm-up exercise for both client and practitioner. Reflexology is not considered massage therapy, therefore, there are no prerequisites for this class.